essential oils and aromatics

a step-by-step guide for use in
massage and aromatherapy

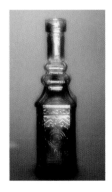

marge clark

SILVERLEAF
PRESS

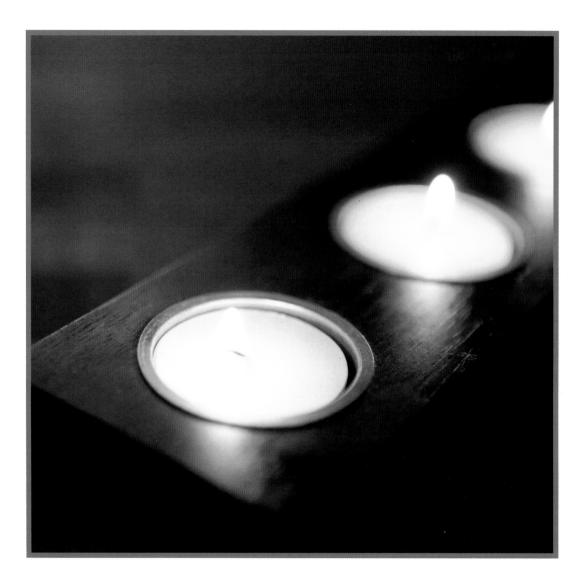

contents

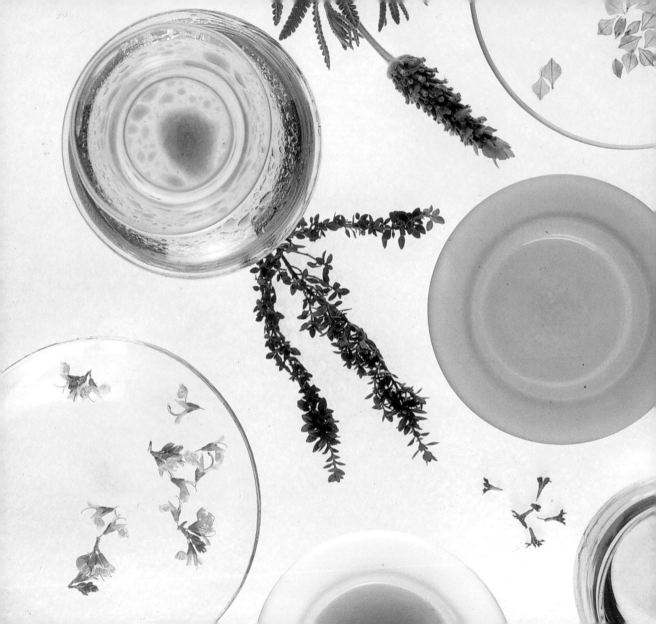

Introduction

My introduction to aromatherapy came from searching for a lovely natural aroma. Years ago I purchased a bottle of lavender essential oil to "boost" the scent of a potpourri blend. Curious, as usual, I researched the lavender oil to see what else it could be used for. I was a bit skeptical, until the first time a friend had a headache. I put a drop on her temples and the back of her neck, and within a few minutes the headache was gone. Then I burned my hand in the oven. I found lavender helped! From there I researched other oils with the few books on the subject available in the '80s, and I was hopelessly hooked. I started giving blends to friends, who kept requesting more, which led to sourcing a larger variety and higher quality of oils. At that point, I started selling what I had in order to buy more.

Founding Nature's Gift (www.naturesgift.com) exposed me to clients all over the world who continually send feedback on ways the oils have made a difference in the quality of their lives. I continue to be in awe of the healing power of these oils, and have used the website to teach about their safe and appropriate use. Almost daily I hear from clients who have had physical or emotional pain eased by using the correct essential oils. This book seemed a natural outgrowth of these earlier activities.

My daughter once described what we do in these words, "Every day, all over the world, we send out boxes full of joy and healing." I hope readers of this book will find their own paths to joy and healing in its pages.

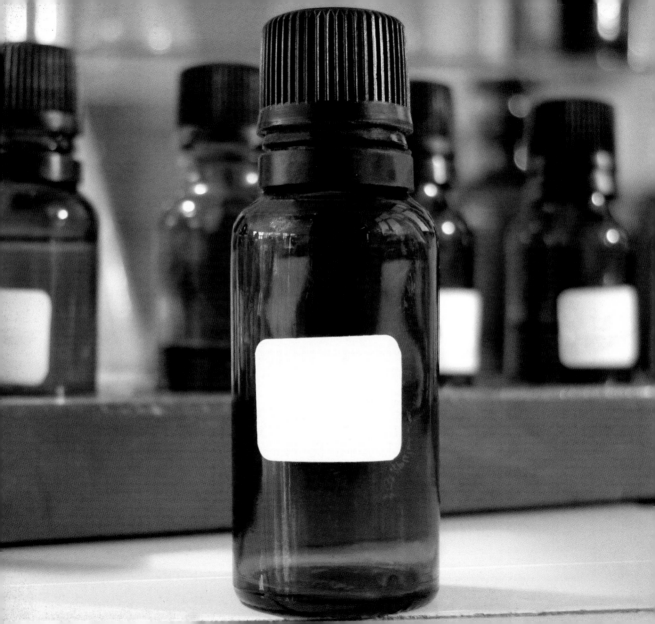

Essential Oils

Pure essential oils are the most powerful form of a healing plant. The term "essential oil" is, perhaps, a misnomer. The precious essential oils are not, in fact, "oily," but rather very volatile substances. When you pick a fresh herb and bruise a leaf, the aroma you smell is the essential oil being released from scent glands in the leaf. The scent of your grandmother's cedar chest comes from the essential oil of the cedarwood it is lined with. The scent of incense burned in a cathedral comes from the essential oil in the frankincense resin. The "bouquet of roses" comes from the essential oil in the rose petals.

The unique thing about essential oils is that when inhaled they both are absorbed into the bloodstream and have a direct effect on the brain. In the bloodstream, the aromatic molecules of essential oils interact with the body's chemistry. This is why essential oils can be used to heal the body as well as uplift the spirits. Many aromatherapists practice the art of using essential oils to enhance moods and emotions as well as easing pain and combatting infections.

True essential oils are steam distilled from roots (e.g., vetiver, ginger), wood (e.g., sandalwood, cedarwood), resins (e.g., frankincense, myrrh), berries (juniper), flowers (e.g., lavender, rose), or leaves (e.g., rosemary, lemongrass, tea tree).

quality

How do I know that I am buying a high quality essential oil? Are they all the same quality? How do I tell a good essential oil from a mediocre or a synthetic one? And does it matter?

For those of us using the essential oils for psychological and emotional nurturing and for their therapeutic benefits, quality matters immensely. Most essential oils are produced for the food and flavoring industry or for commercial perfumers. These industries demand that the essential oils they use are identical, year after year. This is easy for a chemist to do. The essential oil may be adjusted by removing some of the naturally occurring plant chemicals or by adding other chemicals, natural or synthetic, to match a certain profile. These may still be termed, and marketed, as "essential oils," but they are not what we want for aromatherapy.

the methods of producing essential oils

Steam distillation
Hydrodistillation
Water and steam distillation
Cold pressing
Solvent extraction
Carbon dioxide extraction

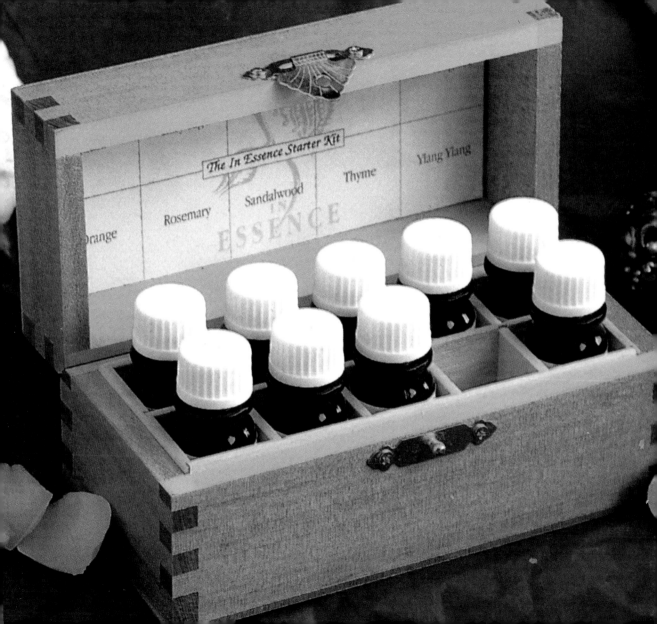

As a consumer, there are some things to look for on the bottles of essential oil that you purchase.

1. They should be bottled in colored glass, usually amber, cobalt, violet, or green. Exposure to sunlight damages the essential oils, so they need to be stored in colored glass.
2. The bottles should never be offered with "eye dropper" bottle tops. The essential oils are powerful solvents and can melt the rubber stopper of the dropper top.
3. The label should give you specific information.
    a. the "common name" (e.g., lavender)
    b. the botanical species (e.g., *Lavandula angustifolia*) (There is more than one species of lavender.)
    c. the country of origin (e.g., Bulgaria, France, India) (Lavender essential oil is produced in all of these countries. There is extreme variance between countries.)
    d. the plant part distilled (e.g., blossom, root, leaf) (Some plants yield essential oil from more than one part. Examples are cinnamon leaf and bark, or angelica root and seed.)
    e. the method of cultivation (e.g., organic farming, conventional farming, wild crafting)
    f. the method of production (e.g., steam distillation, cold pressing) (There is a huge difference, aromatically, between rose absolute and rose essential oil. Which is "better" depends on the proposed use.)
4. Prices will vary widely. Some essential oils are relatively low-priced because their plants of origin are comparably easy to grow and they yield a tremendous amount of essential oil. Examples of relatively low-priced essential oils are some of the cold pressed citrus oils, eucalyptus, lemongrass, and peppermint. Medium-priced oils will include rosemary, clary sage, and frankincense. The "precious oils," both rare and costly, will include rose, sandalwood, and *Helichrysum Italicuum*. Beware of any shop offering peppermint and rose at anywhere near the same price.
5. Samples. Are samples available? Does the supplier offer more than one type of "the same" oil, i.e., different varieties? I would never buy an essential oil without first sampling it, unless it was from a source I knew and trusted. Does the sample smell clean, fresh, and vibrant? Remember, not every essential oil smells "pretty."
6. Does the supplier seem knowledgeable about the oils they sell? Are they familiar with the uses of that particular oil and any safety issues about its uses?

This is the absolute minimum that should be on the label. A reputable supplier will know the provenance of his or her oils and will most likely be glad to share the information.

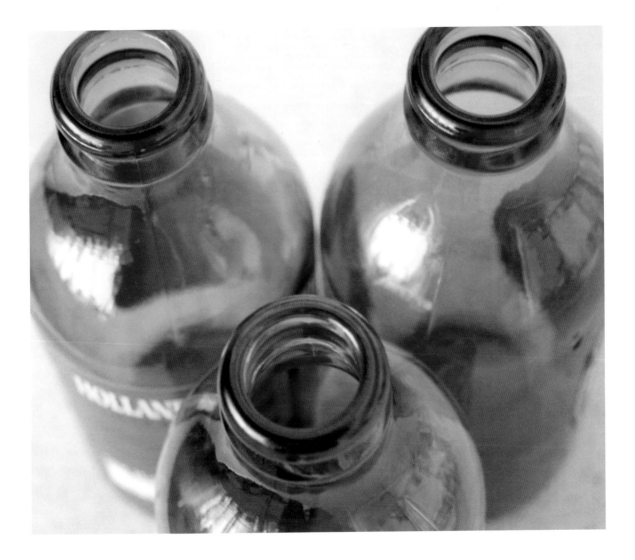

storage

Now that I have them, how do I store them? Most essential oils do best when stored, tightly sealed, at a cool room temperature, away from heat and light. A cool cabinet or drawer is best. Don't store them near a source of heat or on a sunny windowsill. Some essential oils, primarily the cold pressed citrus oils and the conifers (needle oils: fir, pine, spruce, etc.), should be refrigerated if they are not used daily. Air, as well as heat and bright lights, can damage the more fragile oils. Keep the bottles tightly sealed, and as you empty a bottle, decant the remaining essential oil in a smaller bottle. A full bottle doesn't leave room for air. It is the oxygen in the air that damages the essential oil.

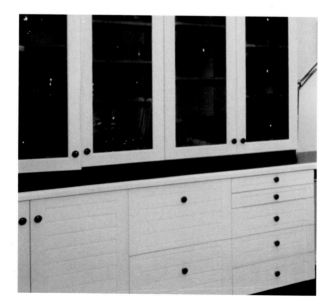

essential oil notes

The depth or weight of a specific essential oil's aroma is based on the oil's volatility, how fast it evaporates. Essential oils are classified into three categories according to the rate at which they evaporate—or how long their fragrance will last—relative to other oils. These categories are "top note," "middle note," and "base note."

As a general rule of thumb, the top notes are citrus rind oils (lemon, orange, mandarine), conifers (pine, spruce, fir), and some very light florals (champa, orange blossom). Heart notes tend to be most florals (lavender, neroli, jasmine), most herbs (sweet marjoram, clary sage) and grasses. Base notes tend to be woods and roots.

There are exceptions to this rule. Rose is a very deep floral and tends to be categorized as a "low heart" note. Patchouli, although a grass, is a very powerful base note. Lemongrass, although a grass and presumably a heart note is either a top note, or, at most, a high heart note. I have seen peppermint classified in all three categories; perhaps it depends on what else it is being blended with.

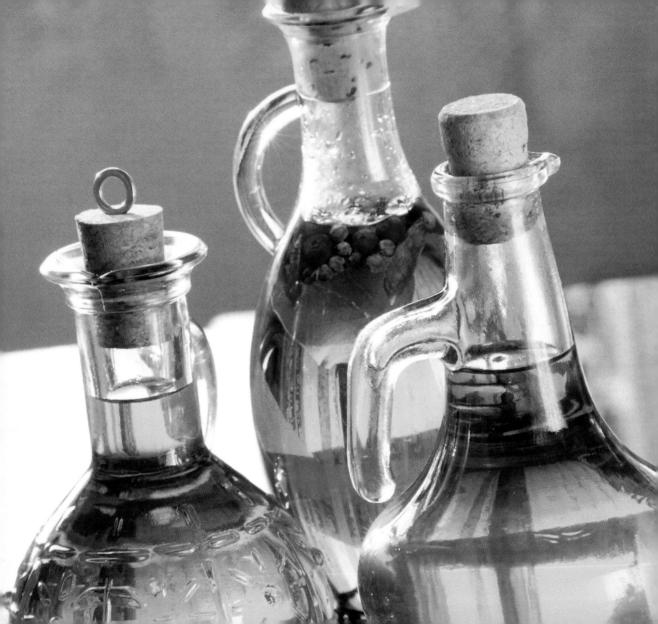

Carrier Oils

No essential oil should be used undiluted ("neat") on the skin. For this reason, we use the fixed, vegetable oils to dilute them. These are called carrier oils. Essential oils are oil soluble (will dissolve in a carrier oil) while they will not dissolve in water. Some carrier oils have their own health or skin care benefits.

When possible, please choose your carrier oils as carefully as you do your much more costly essential oils. Choose the cold pressed, rather than solvent extracted, and organically grown, if available. Please note when I suggest using the carrier oil in a certain percentage, that means that if blending carrier oils, you will want to use at least that much in your total blend to receive the benefits of that oil. Blending oil is helpful because some may have a texture that is too thick or heavy for you. Blending oils also cuts costs by mixing less expensive oils with more expensive oils.

some commonly available carrier oils and their qualities include:

almond oil/sweet almond oil

Helpful to all skin types. Especially good for eczema. Helps relieve itching, soreness, dryness, and inflammation. Useful against burns and thread veins. Very lubricating, but not penetrating—this makes it a good massage oil and protectant. Goes rancid fairly quickly.

apricot kernel oil

For all skin types. Very rich and nourishing. Helpful for prematurely aged, sensitive, inflamed, delicate, or dry skin. Can be used 100% strength, but normally used at 10–50%. Apricot kernel oil is clear and light in texture, one of my favorites for mature skin. I use it as the primary base oil in all my skin care applications.

avocado oil

Very penetrating. Nourishing for dry and dehydrated skin, eczema, solar keratosis. Improves elasticity. Very thick heavy oil, best blended with others. Normally used at 10% dilution.

borage seed oil

Used internally used for PMT, MS, and menopausal problems, heart disease. Used externally for psoriasis, eczema, prematurely aged skin; it is also good for regenerating and stimulating skin cell activity. Very penetrating. Goes rancid very quickly. Use at 10% dilution.

calophyllum (foraha or tamanu)

This exotic and unusual green carrier, cold pressed from the berry of a shrub that grows in Madagascar, is believed to have pain relieving effects, making it useful for rheumatism, arthritis, sciatica, etc. Useful for lesions due to herpes and/or shingles (especially when combined with *Ravensara Aromatica* essential oil). Sometimes recommended for treatment of physical and chemical burns.

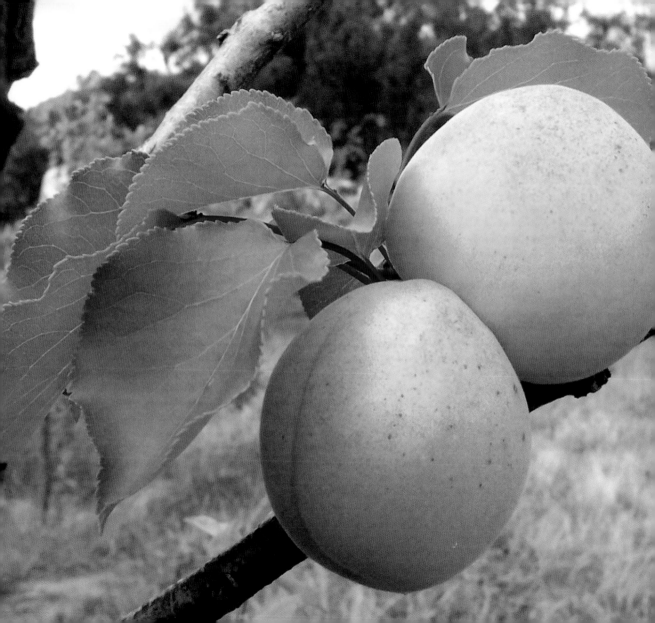

The oil may be used as a base oil or an additive. Be careful on sensitive skin, it can be an irritant. If using it for skin care, my instinct would be to use it at perhaps 10–25% of the total carrier oils.

Some sources recommend calophyllum for cellular regeneration, saying it is a powerful healer for burns, cuts, etc. It may also help with eczema, burns, rashes, and insect bites. I have seen it recommended in skin care blends for mature skin and to help relieve eczema.

fractionated coconut oil

Not a truly "natural" oil, fractionated coconut is the light, liquid portion of normally solid coconut oil. It is as clear as water, a very light liquid. Fractionated coconut oil has many advantages; one is its virtually unlimited shelf life. Since it doesn't turn rancid or clog pores, it is an ideal carrier for oily or troubled skin. Its long shelf life also makes it the perfect diluent for the more costly essential oils. Another advantage for the massage therapist: fractionated coconut oil will easily wash out of linens in the laundry, unlike most cold pressed vegetable oils. Used for dryness, itching, sensitive skin, and as a tanning aid. Use as base or 10–50% additive. Adding to sweet almond oil increases both shelf life and "washability."

evening primrose oil

Internally used for premenstrual tension, multiple sclerosis, and menopausal problems. Externally for psoriasis, and eczema. Helps to prevent prematurely aged skin and aids in healing wounds and scars. Primrose has a very short shelf life.

grapeseed oil

Best for oily skin, odorless, and penetrating. A very light oil. Slightly astringent, it tightens and tones the skin. Does not aggravate acne. Use full strength. Grapeseed oil is solvent extracted. It is a useful oil for massage since it is not quickly absorbed.

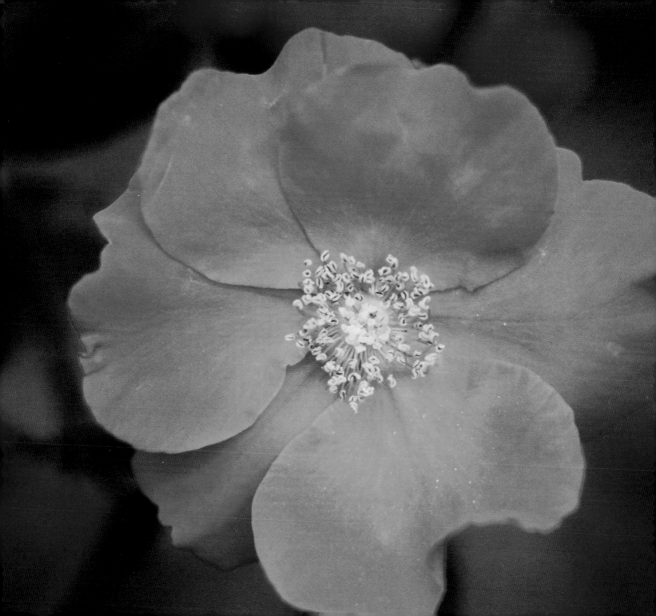

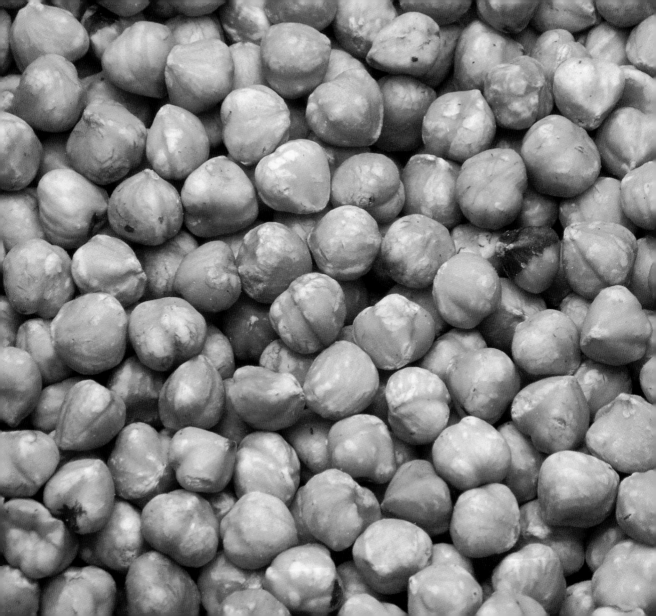

hazelnut oil

Excellent oil for oily skin, slightly astringent, toning, with a fast absorption. Useful as base for oily, combination skins, and for acne. Tones and tightens skin, helps maintain firmness and elasticity. Helps to strengthen capillaries, so it might be useful against thread veins. Hazelnut encourages cell regeneration and stimulates circulation. Use 100% as base or in 10% dilution.

jojoba oil

This is actually a liquid wax. Mimics sebum, penetrates skin rapidly, therefore not necessarily a good massage oil, but excellent for nourishing skin. May help extend the life of other oils. Healing for inflamed skins, psoriasis, eczema, any sort of dermatitis. Can help control acne and oily skin or scalp since excess sebum actually dissolves in jojoba. Antioxidant, used also for hair care. Useful for all skin types. Can clog pores. Myristic acid is anti-inflammatory, so this could be a good base oil for treating rheumatism and arthritis. Use as 10% dilution or full strength. Jojoba oil is one of my favorite carriers for diluting blends and for a basic skin care oil.

kukui nut oil

Extremely good penetration to all skin levels, soothes irritation, sunburn, lesions, and burns. Protects tissue from drying. Cosmetic chemists report that kukui oil has an excellent skin feel. They say the kukui oil seems to be readily absorbed into the skin (it does not leave a greasy film). Kukui nut oil seems to make chapped or rough, dry skin feel smooth, silky, and soft. Is said to prevent scarring when applied to abrasions. Use as 5–10% additive.

macadamia nut oil

All skin types. Tones aged or dry skin. Skin-softening, wound healing. In France macadamia nut oil is used as an aid against sunburn. Macadamia's fatty acids are helpful in maintaining the skin's critical water barrier functions. It is self-stabilizing and requires no antioxidants. In addition, it has an excellent safety profile that includes low order of oral toxicity. All of this suggests its usefulness in facial products, baby products, balms, and lip glosses.

olive oil

Useful for rheumatic conditions, hair care, cosmetics, soothing, nail, and hair care. Helpful for inflamed skin, acne, bruises, and sprains. Strong odor makes it more useful with strongly scented essential oils. Use 10–50% dilution. Traditionally used to produce macerated oils. Please use only virgin olive oil or extra virgin (from the first pressing). Lower grades may contain solvents.

rose hip seed oil

Useful for dry, scaly, fissured skin, dull skin, eczema, psoriasis, over-pigmented skin, scars. Blend with *Helichrysum Italicum* for fading old scars. Prophylactic after burns or trauma. Good for ulcerated veins and scars. Avoid with acne and oily or blemished skins. Use as 10% additive or neat for very dry, aging skins. Goes rancid very quickly. Rose hip seed is the perfect carrier oil for anti-aging skin care blends.

squalane

Like rose hip seed oil, squalane is a "specialty oil" but well worth the trouble to seek out. This all-vegetable product, extracted from olive oil, is one of the most powerful moisturizers I have encountered. Clear and colorless, it looks like water in the bottle. Research shows that squalane not only moisturizes the skin, but also provides a barrier preventing transdermal water loss. It is an ideal ingredient in any blend for dry, chapped, or scaly skin. I have heard excellent reports from people using it in salves and balms to help ease the discomfort of eczema or contact dermatitis.

Squalane is a natural component of human skin during childhood and adolescence, but as we enter our twenties, the amount present decreases rapidly, contributing to the aging process. Will adding a drop of squalane to your normal skin care regime give you the glowing complexion of a child? I doubt it! But it should restore moisture and suppleness. I would avoid using on oily or acne-prone skin.

sunflower oil

Prophylactic to all skin types, used to treat leg ulcers and skin diseases, bruises, diaper rash, and cradle cap. Easily absorbed. Light textured.

dilution and equivalents for carrier oils

Measurements/conversions (volume)

30 mL	I fl oz	600 drops	2 tablespoonfuls
15 mL	1/2 fl oz	300 drops	I tablespoonful
5 mL	1/6 fl oz	100 drops	I teaspoon
I mL	1/30 fl oz	20 drops	1/5 teaspoon

How to achieve a specific dilution

For one fluid ounce of carrier oil:

I% of 600 drops (I fl oz) =	6 drops
2% of 600 drops (I fl oz) =	12 drops
2.5% of 600 drops (I fl oz) =	15 drops
5% of 600 drops (I fl oz) =	30 drops
10% of 600 drops (I fl oz) =	60 drops

Using Essential Oils

Essential oils can be used in several different ways. Try some lavender essential oil in a cool compress to ease a headache. Or mix bergamot essential oil into a spritzer and spray the blend into a room that needs a little freshening up. Once you learn the methods, you can become creative in how you use your favorite essential oils.

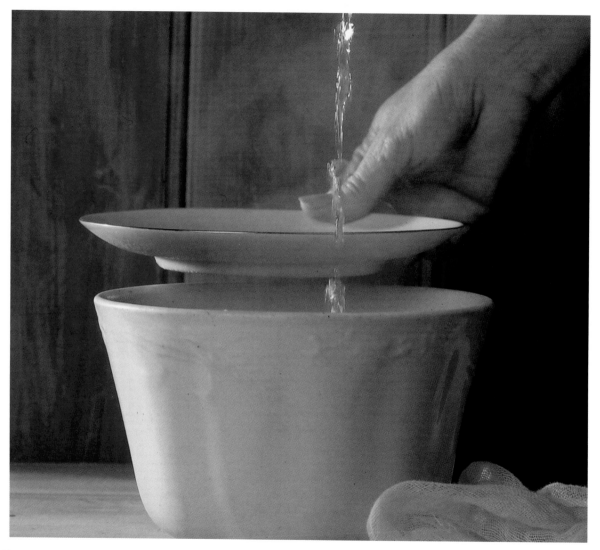

compresses

Excellent for topical application to ease the pain of strained muscles, menstrual cramps, and more. Add 4–7 drops of essential oil to a bowl of warm water. Swish the surface of the water with a cloth, wring out, and apply to affected area. Repeat when the cloth cools. You may cover the warm cloth with a sheet of plastic and a towel to keep the warmth in longer. This is an excellent method for treating painful menstrual cramps. Compresses may be either warm (to ease cramping or lower back pain) or cool (to ease a headache or a sprain).

inhalation

The easiest form of inhalation is to simply put a drop of the appropriate essential oil or blend on a tissue and inhale. A drop of lavender on your pillowcase will ease you to sleep on a restless night.

When you don't wish to fill the room or your house with the oils you are using, simply fill a bowl or small sink with hot water, add 6–8 drops of essential oil, and put a towel over your head and the bowl. Inhale slowly and deeply, keeping the eyes closed. This is a wonderful method for combating a head cold or bronchial congestion. Please avoid this method when dealing with asthma.

diffusers

The most common diffusers are aroma lamps, sometimes called potpourri pots or burners. A ceramic or glass bowl sits over a tea candle. Fill the bowl with warm water, add 6–8 drops of essential oil or blend. Light the tea candle under the bowl. The water vapor will disperse throughout the room, carrying the essential oil with it. For emotional benefits or simply for ambience, an attractive aroma lamp has a delightful effect.

There are also various styles of electric diffusers available. Some contain a fan and a pad of cellulose. Moisten the pad with your chosen essential oil, turn on the fan, and a stream of cool air will disperse the oil. Some, called nebulizers, contain ornate blown glass fittings that hold a small amount of essential oil. Air is blown through the nebulizer from a pump similar to an aquarium pump. The essential oil is sprayed into the air in microscopic particles, capable of staying in the air for up to two hours. This is probably one of the most effective methods of diffusion for therapeutic benefits. There is one drawback, however. I have never found a nebulizer with a silent air pump.

New to the aromatherapy products market is a "Cool Mist" humidifier, especially designed to add humidity to the air along with the precious essential oils. Diffusers are available to plug into your car to keep the air fresh for driver and passengers.

Not recommended for use are the so-called "lamp rings" that sit on a light bulb. It's my experience that they tend to "burn" the fragile essential oils, rather than dispersing them.

topical application

Whenever a diluted essential oil is applied directly to the skin, you are using it "topically." Please note the word "diluted" above. Essential oils should never be applied "neat," or undiluted, to the skin. (Proper dilution, and a dilution table, is given on page 23)

sprays or spritzers

The amount of essential oil used depends on the purpose of the spritzer. To 4 ounces of distilled water add:

- 8–10 drops for a facial toner
- 30–40 drops for an all over body spritzer
- 80–100 drops for a room spray/air freshener or linen spray

Shake well, spray. May be used as a facial toner, to moisten a body wrap, as an all over freshener,

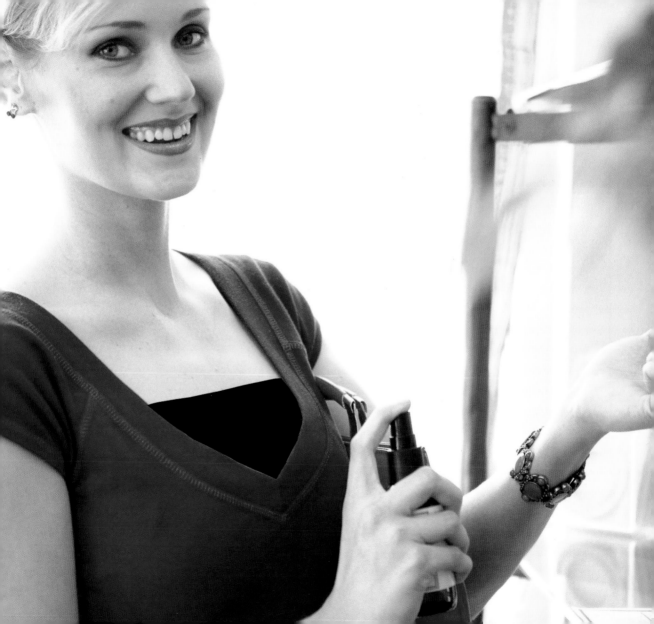

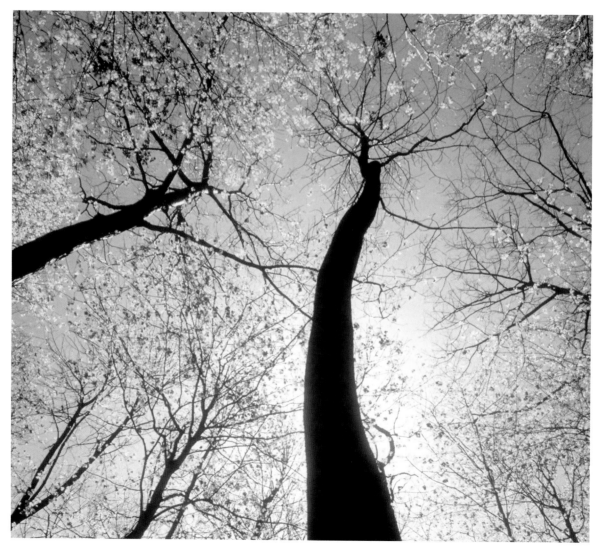

Safety Concerns

The Greek "pharmakon" means both medicine and poison, because anything powerful enough to heal is powerful enough to do damage. Some of the most beneficial oils can prove harmful under certain conditions. Concentrated oils are very strong. Just because a product is natural doesn't mean that it's harmless. After all, poison ivy is totally natural. Inappropriate use of essential oils can often lead to adverse and damaging side effects.

photosensitivity

Some oils have the likelihood of causing severe and permanent skin damage if they are applied to skin that is likely to be exposed to sunlight or ultraviolet light. These oils should never be used in any product that will be left on the skin.

Highest risk: bergamot, expressed lime (not steam distilled), rue, cumin, angelica, caraway, cassia, and cinnamon bark. Please note that a "sunsafe" version of bergamot is available. Commonly known as bergamot FCF, it has the Bergaptene removed.

Moderate risk: lemon, St. John's Wort infused oil, and grapefruit

Slight risk: mandarin, tangerine, orange, patchouli, and petitgrain (very mild)

irritation

This is the most common type of reaction, and is characterized by various degrees of dermal inflammation. The reaction is localized and does not involve the immune system. Many essential oils are skin irritants, even in relatively low dilutions. Almost any essential oil has the potential to irritate the skin if not diluted enough. Remember, less is more when dealing with these powerful extracts.

allergic sensitivity

This is also known as contact allergic or sensitivity reaction. This is an immune system reaction. To start this type of reaction, first the substance has to enter the skin, bind with lymphatic tissues, and then cause the T cells to become sensitized. If, at any time in the future, the same substance or a chemically-related substance is once more introduced to the skin or possibly any other part of the body, the immune system will react to this substance perceiving it as a threat and cause a severe, possibly life-threatening reaction. The resulting rash may be blotchier than with irritation. The reaction may be much quicker and severe in nature, possibly leading to ana-phylaxis unless quick treatment with adrenalin or antihistamines is available.

One of my mentors reminds me "sensitization is forever." And I know she is right. Years ago I read the books saying that lavender oil could be used neat (undiluted). I very unwisely used un-diluted lavender on broken skin, and consequently set up a sensitivity reaction. Today, almost two decades later, if I come in contact with lavender in any form, I will immediately start a new round of contact dermatitis that can take months to heal.

Sensitization can happen at random, however some essential oils and absolutes are known sen-sitizers and should never be used on the skin.

Essential oils with a proven history of causing sensitization (allergies): benzoin (indeed, any sty-rax oil), Peru balsam, calamus, cassia, cinnamon bark and leaf, costus, fig leaf absolute, galbanum resin (cross sensitizing with Peru balsam), tolu (balsam, very strong) and lemon verbena (the International Fragrance Research Association strongly advises against the use of verbena oil in cosmetics or perfume products).

Many other essential oils are suspected of having the potential to create a sensitization reaction, so use all oils in a mild dilution for your own safety. Individuals with a history of allergies, asthma, or ec-zema are more prone to developing a sensitization reaction and will need to exercise extra caution.

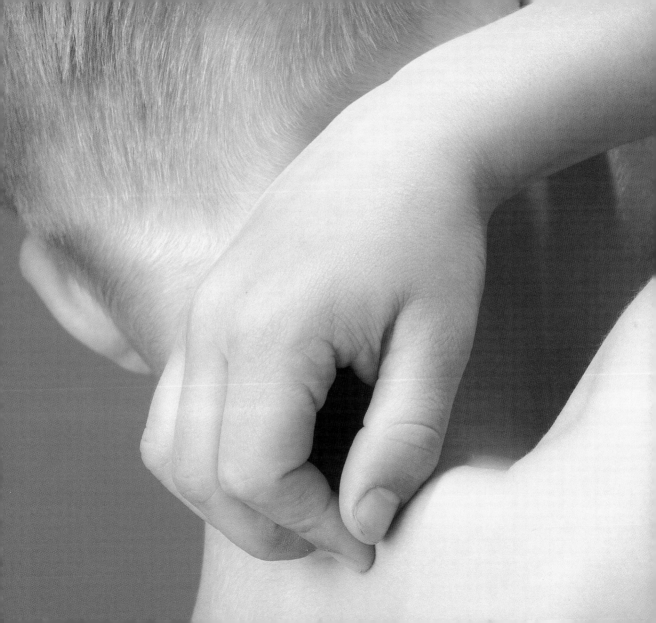

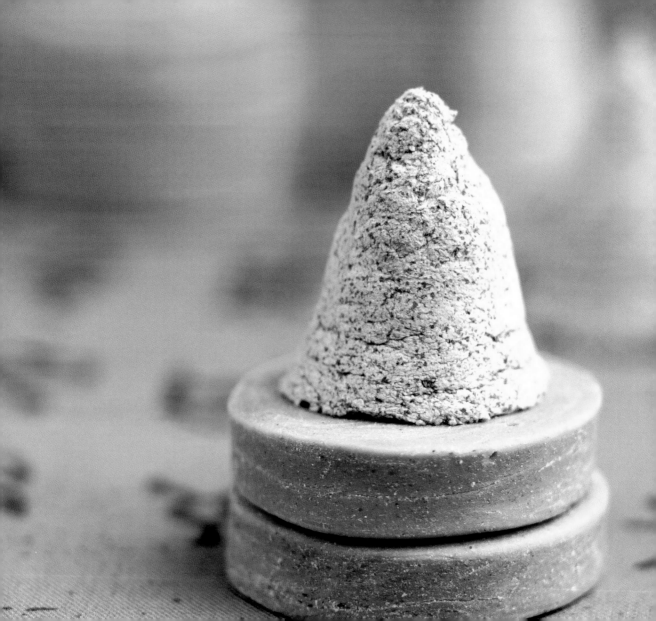

The Art of Aromatherapy

The healing art of aromatherapy has been defined as "altering the body or the emotions by the safe and appropriate use of pure essential oils." True aromatherapy can have powerful effects both physically and emotionally. Carefully chosen essential oils used appropriately can ease a headache, calm a fretful toddler, soothe an insomniac into peaceful sleep, clear congested sinuses, relieve the pain of sore muscles, kill household germs, and even allay anxiety. Plus, it smells wonderful!

Aromatherapy does not, as practiced in North America, normally include the internal use of essential oils. It does not use synthetic "fragrance oils" such as mango, peach, rain, or applejack, but true natural aromatics of botanical origin.

Botanical medicine has been practiced since the beginning of time. Our forefathers (or foremothers?) knew that simmering the appropriate herb into tea could ease a fever, and that a poultice of certain herbs could ease pain. The ancient Egyptians, Romans, Tibetans, and Native Americans (as well as all other early civilizations) infused oils and fats with rare resins and aromatic plants to produce healing unguents. They also used the smoke of burning herbs and produced teas and tisanes from healing plants. The use of nature's bounty for healing and for sacred rituals is as old as mankind.

The discovery of penicillin and other "wonder drugs" left botanical medicine in the shadows for decades. Today, with the emergence of "super bugs," resistant to many of our familiar antibacterial medicines, the essential oils have a long forgotten role to play. Because every essential oil differs slightly, even when distilled from the same plants, bacteria cannot develop the resistance that renders our laboratory-produced medicines ineffective. Just as no two snowflakes are identical, neither are two pure, natural essential oils.

Please note that aromatherapy is a complimentary modality and is not meant to replace conventional medical treatment. However, it does provide a way to both supplement conventional medical treatment and allow the user to practice self-care and self-nurturing. No suggestions in this book are intended to replace your healthcare provider.

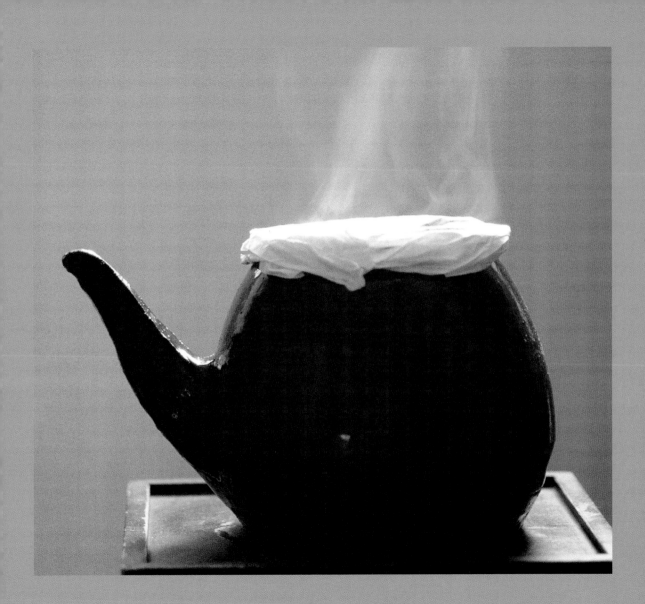

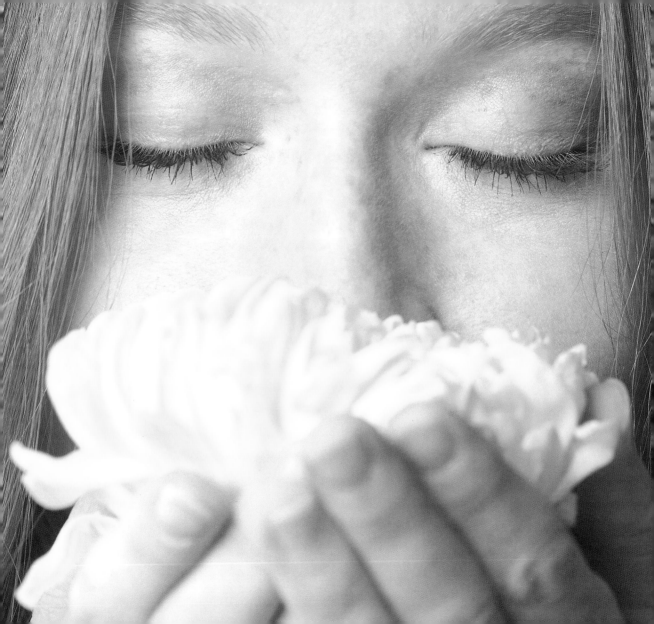

Aromatherapy for Mind and Mood

Had a frustrating day at work? Try a bath of chamomile to relax your anger. Nervous for an upcoming wedding? Diffuse a little neroli in a room freshener to calm your emotions. And if you are just feeling a little blue, add some jasmine or citrus to your body spritzer—you'll be feeling uplifted in no time. Essential oils have long been known to enhance moods and lighten the spirits. Take advantage of these natural solutions and make your life a little more livable.

emotional uses

To Ease:	Try:
Anger	chamomile, jasmine, marjoram, palma rosa, rose, rosemary, ylang-ylang
Anxiety	neroli, bergamot, Roman chamomile, frankincense, geranium (for balance), lavender, orange, patchouli, rose (for confidence), sandalwood, sweet marjoram, vetiver (for grounding)
Disappointment	bergamot, cypress, frankincense, jasmine, orange, rose
Fear	cedarwood, fennel, ginger, patchouli, sandalwood, spikenard, thyme
Grief	bergamot, chamomile, jasmine, marjoram, neroli, rose
Hysteria	Roman chamomile, lavender, neroli, orange, tea tree, vetiver
Impatience	chamomile, clary, frankincense, lavender
Indecision	basil, clary, cypress, jasmine, lemon, patchouli, peppermint
Jealousy	jasmine, rose
Loneliness	benzoin, marjoram
Fatigue (emotional and mental)	basil, clary, cardamon, cinnamon leaf or bark, clove bud, coriander, eucalyptus citriodora, ginger, grapefruit, helichrysum, jasmine, juniper, orange, palmarosa, peppermint, rosemary, thyme, vetiver, ylang-ylang
Fatigue (physical)	basil, elemi, ginger, lemon, lavender, orange, peppermint, rosemary
Nervousness	chamomile, clary, coriander, frankincense, neroli, orange, vetiver
Panic	chamomile, clary, geranium, jasmine, juniper, lavender, neroli, ylang-ylang
Sadness	benzoin, jasmine, rose, rosewood
Shyness	black pepper, ginger, jasmine, patchouli, peppermint, rose, neroli, ylang-ylang
Stress	bergamot, 'Atlas' cedarwood, Roman chamomile, all citrus oils, clary sage, frank-incense, geranium, lavender, sweet marjoram, melissa, neroli, patchouli, petitgrain, rose (absolute and otto), rosemary, sandalwood, vetiver, ylang-ylang
Suspicion	jasmine, lavender
Tension	chamomile, clary, cypress, frankincense, geranium, jasmine, lavender, lemon, marjoram, neroli, orange, rose, rosewood, sandalwood, ylang-ylang

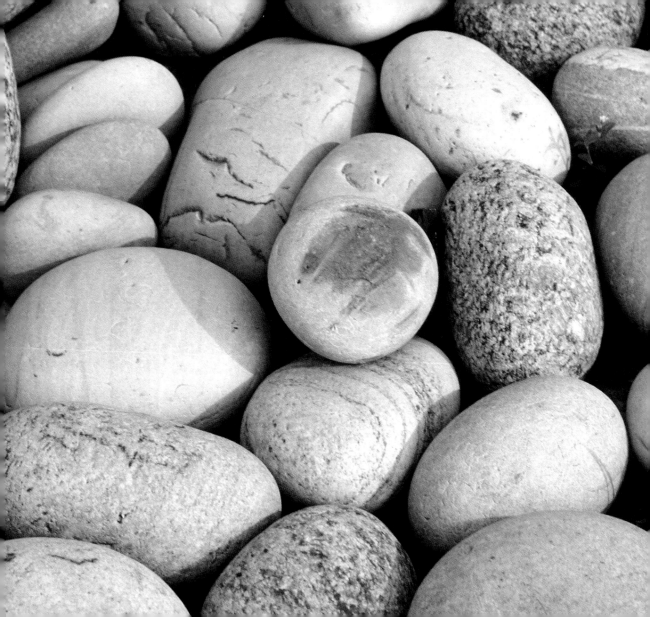

essential oil effects

Basil: uplifting, refreshing, clarifying, aids concentration
Bergamot: refreshing, uplifting
Chamomile (Roman): refreshing, relaxing, soothing, anti-inflammatory
Cedarwood: relaxing, calming, soothing, strengthening
Clary sage: warming, relaxing, uplifting, calming, euphoric
Cypress: relaxing, refreshing, astringent
Eucalyptus: head clearing, antiseptic, decongestant, invigorating
Fennel: carminative, eases wind and indigestion, mild diuretic
Frankincense: relaxing, eases breathing, dispels fears, spiritually uplifting
Geranium: refreshing, relaxing, balancing, harmonizing
Hyssop: decongestant
Jasmine: relaxing, soothing, confidence building, aphrodisiac
Juniper: refreshing, stimulating, relaxing, diuretic
Lavender: refreshing, relaxing, therapeutic, calming, soothing
Lemon: refreshing, stimulating, uplifting, motivating
Lemongrass: toning, refreshing, fortifying
Marjoram: warming, fortifying, sedating
Melissa: uplifting, refreshing, anti-viral
Myrrh: toning, strengthening, rejuvenating, anti-bacterial
Neroli: relaxing, dispels fears, anti-anxiety
Orange: refreshing, relaxing
Peppermint: cooling, refreshing, head clearing
Pine: refreshing, antiseptic, invigorating, stimulating
Rose: relaxing, soothing, sensual, confidence building
Rosemary: invigorating, refreshing, stimulating, clarifying
Sandalwood: relaxing, warming, confidence building, grounding
Tea tree: antiseptic, refreshing, strengthens the immune system
Thyme: antiseptic, refreshing, strengthens the immune system
Ylang-ylang: relaxing, soothing, enhances sensuality

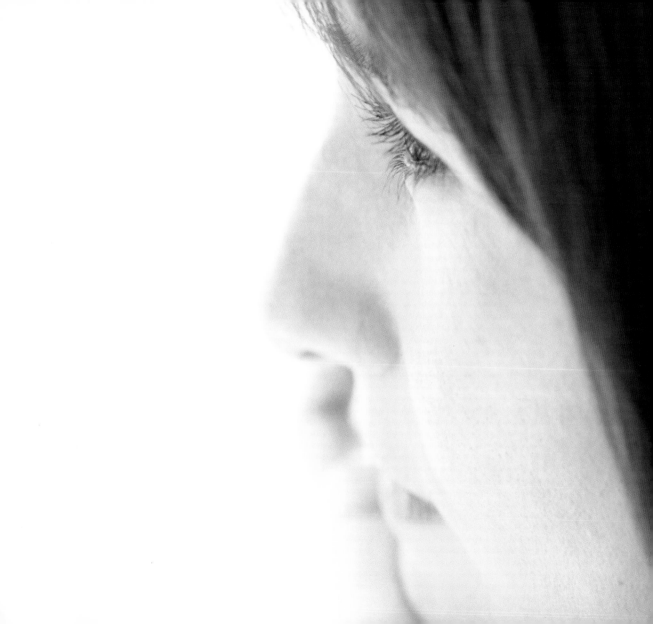

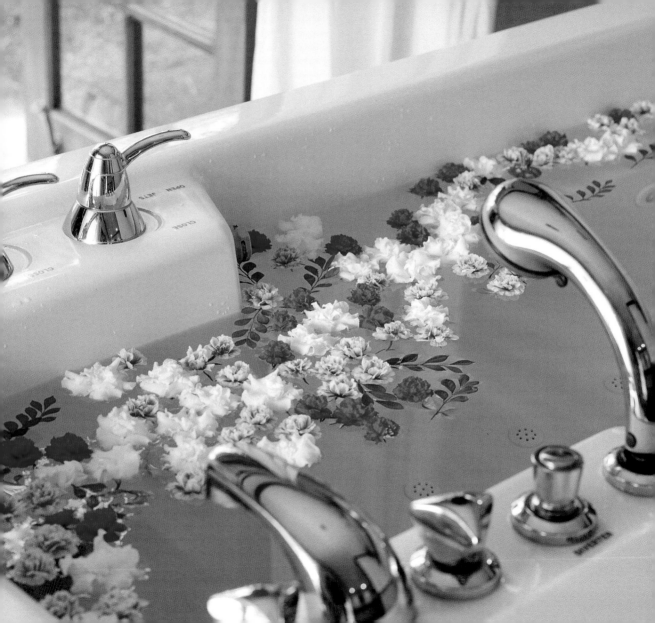

morning wake up shower blend

10 drops peppermint essential oil
5 drops orange essential oil
5 drops spearmint essential oil
3 drops rosemary cineole essential oil

Add 20 drops of the blend to 1 fluid ounce liquid soap or unscented shower gel for a brisk, invigorating morning shower. (This is similar in aroma to a "famous name" salt scrub.)

anxiety reliever

4 drops neroli
2 drops petitgrain
4 drops vetiver
3 drops sandalwood
1 drops frankincense

Blend and use by inhalation. Add 15 drops to your chosen carrier oil and massage. Add 8 drops to a warm bath.

stress reliever bath blend

2 drops lavender
2 drops sandalwood
1 drops Roman chamomile
Or
2 drops geranium
2 drops petitgrain
1 drops neroli

Add 6 to 8 drops of either of the above blends to a soothing bath. Diffusion: black spruce, bergamot, clementine or mandarin. Any of these, in a room diffuser, can relieve stress.

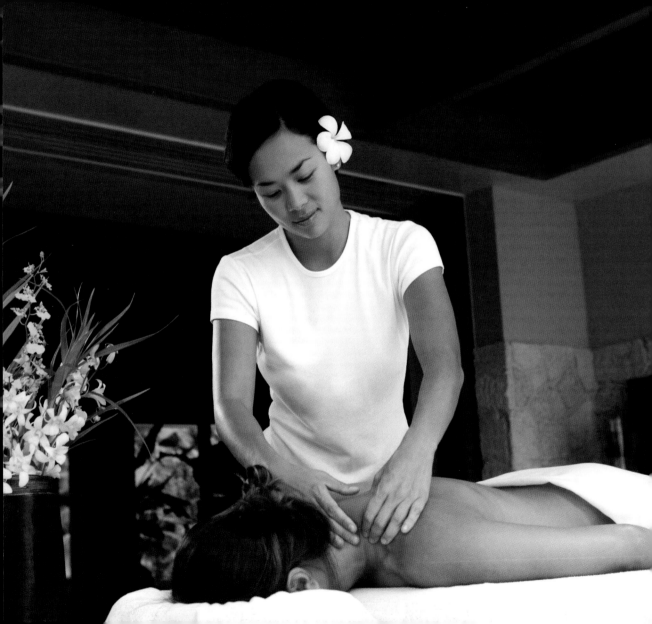

Essential Oils for Massage

Massage is one of the simplest therapeutic treatments. Its physical benefits include stimulating circulation and relaxing tense muscles. Massage also gives an emotional feeling of being cared for and nurtured. When combined with appropriate essential oils, the effects of massage can be truly remarkable.

Essential oils must be diluted before they are applied to the skin. The carrier oil you choose should be pure, have no scent, and be non-sticky so that the hands move easily over the skin. Choose a cold-pressed carrier oil as the properties remain intact.

Many people make a mix and keep the bottle ready for use. Make sure that you don't make more than can be used within the expiration date of the carrier oil. The smell of rancid oil is unappealing. And do not leave the bottle unsealed for any length of time—air accelerates deterioration.

amounts for full body massage

For 1 fluid ounce (30 mL) of carrier oil, use 15–20 drops of essential oil. This gives a 2.5–3% dilution. For children, the frail or elderly, and for pregnant women, the dilution should be a much weaker 1% dilution (⅓ mL or 5–6 drops).

amounts for localized massage

When there is a localized problem, for example a sore shoulder or sprained ankle, use a slightly stronger dilution, just at the affected area. To ½ ounce (15 mL) of carrier oil add 12–15 drops of essential oil or blend. Again, use a much weaker dilution on children or the elderly.

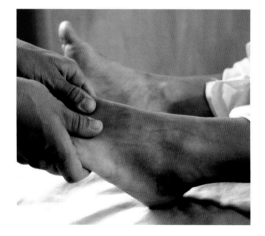

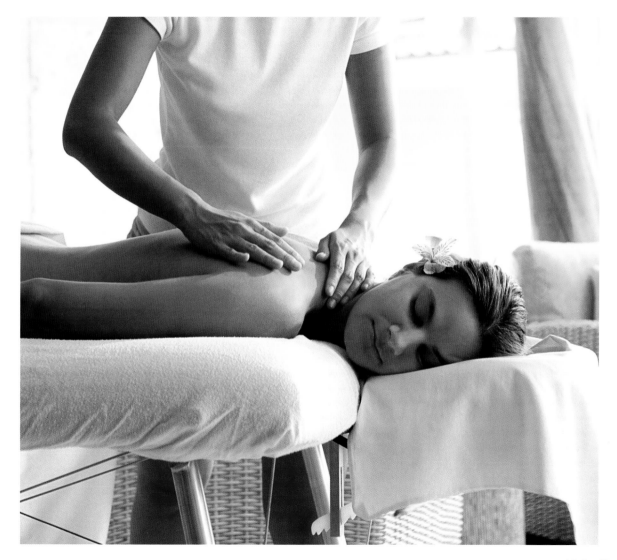

The Aromabath

Both heat and moisture increase the absorption and effectiveness of the oils. Steam and/or warm water vapor also increase the respiratory effects. An aromatic bath is an excellent treatment for overstrained muscles or for frazzled emotions.

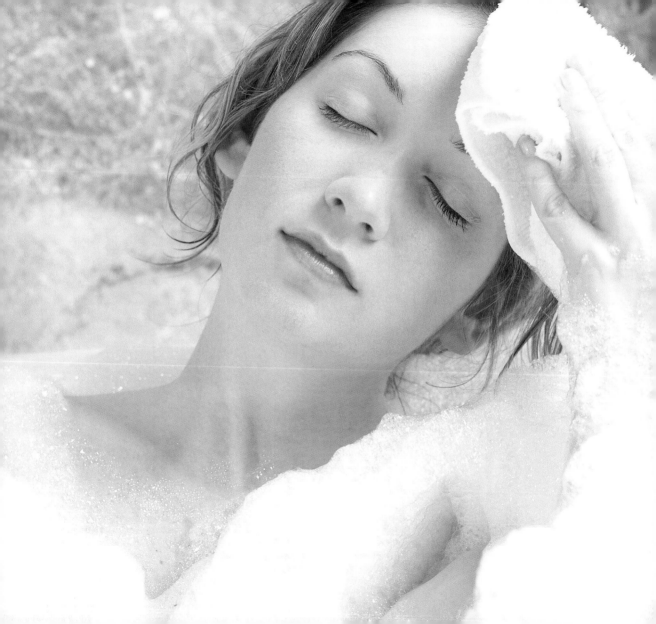

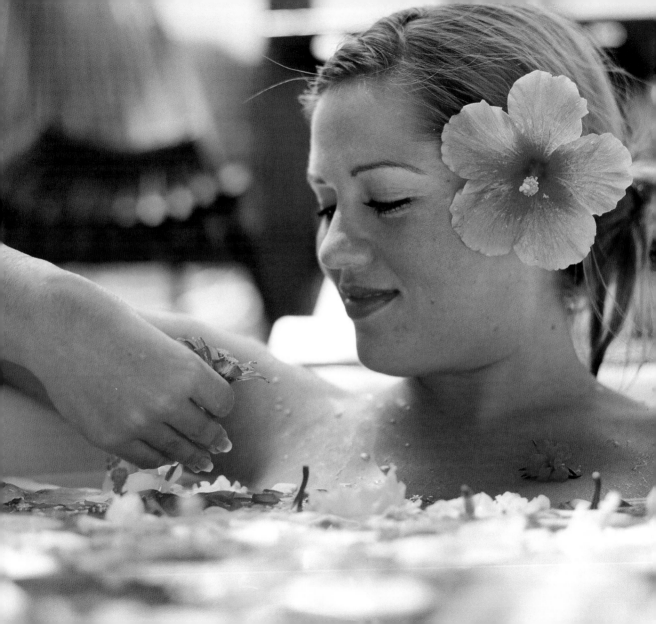

aromatic bath

While running your warm bath, blend 6–12 drops of essential oil into a tablespoon of honey, carrier oil, cream, or milk. Good carrier oils for the bath are sweet almond oil and jojoba oil as they nourish and soften the skin. Swirl into the warm water immediately before entering the tub.

balancing
2 drops geranium
2 drops neroli
2 drops rose

relaxing
2 drops lavender
2 drops bergamot
2 drops cedarwood

revitalizing
3 drops rosemary
2 drops lemon
2 drops frankincense

cleansing and refreshing
3 drops lemon
3 drops geranium

restorative
4 drops lavender
2 drops geranium
2 drops clary sage

shower

Either put a few (4–6) drops of essential oil (or blend) on the floor of the shower when you start running the warm water or, after washing, put 2–3 drops of essential oil on your wet wash cloth and wipe your body down with it. (I prefer the drops on the floor of the shower; the aromatic steam is wonderful.) This is a great method for sleepy mornings when you don't want to get moving. A few drops of an energizing essential oil (pink grapefruit, rosemary, or peppermint) on the shower floor will have you facing the day energized and restored.

jacuzzi/hot tub

Essential oils may be used in the hot tub or Jacuzzi, but don't use a carrier oil to dilute them. Carrier oils will coat or clog the pipes. Just add a few drops of your chosen oil to the water and swish to stir. Avoid using the more irritating oils in any bath.

Healing with Essential Oils

From its appearance in the folk medicine of ancient times, essential oils have been widely recognized for their medicinal properties. Increase your health and well-being with the natural, gentle treatment found in the aromatic compounds of essential oils.

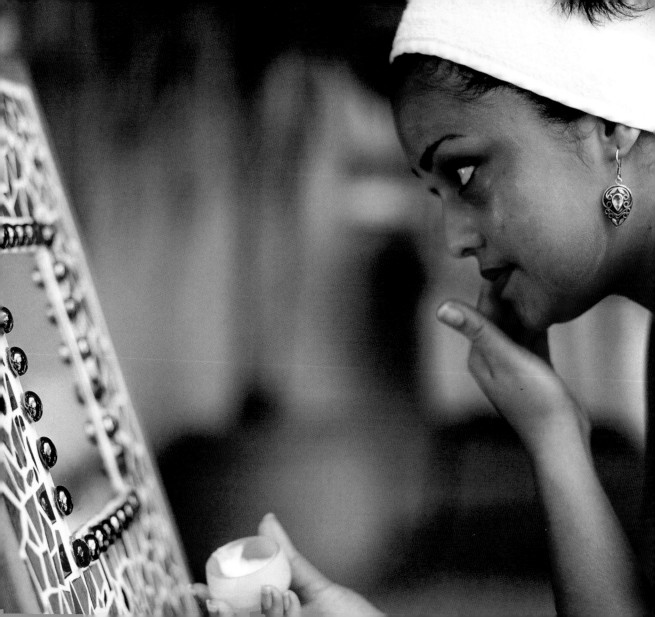

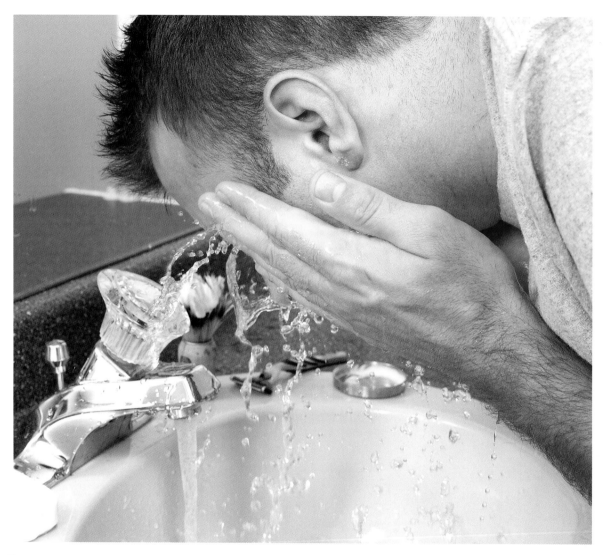

skin care

acne wash
10 drops lavender (antibacterial and soothing)
4 drops manuka or tea tree (antibacterial)
4 drops *German chamomile* (soothing)
4 drops Helichrysum Italicuum (anti-inflammatory and soothing)
10 drops geranium or rose geranium (balancing)

Wash: Add 30 drops of the blend to 1 fluid ounce of liquid castile soap. Rinse well. (This is a strong dilution because it will be washed off.)
Moisturizer: Add 15 drops of the blend to 1 fluid ounce of hazelnut oil. (Hazelnut is mildly astringent and a wonderful choice for oily skin.) If skin is dry, substitute jojoba oil.

mature skin blend
3 drops carrot seed
5 drops frankincense
4 drops sandalwood
3 drops seabuckthorn berry extract
3 drops neroli

Cleanser: Add 15 drops of the above blend to 1 fluid ounce of your favorite unscented cleanser or liquid soap.
Toner: Any of the following hydrosols are wonderful toners for mature skin: cistus, carrot, witch hazel, frankincense, or rose
Moisturizer: Add 10 drops of the above essential oil blend to 1 fluid ounce rose hip seed oil.

scar cream (surgical or burn)

Add 15 drops of *Helichrysum Italicuum* essential oil to one fluid ounce of rose hip seed oil. Apply a small amount to the scar three or four times a day.

basic balm or salve

For winter chapped lips, extra dry or chapped hands, baby's bottom, etc.

Melt together one ounce (by weight, not volume) of beeswax (preferably grated, it will melt faster), a "solid" fat (shea butter is my favorite, but cocoa butter will also work) and one ounce of a rich carrier oil (try jojoba or avocado oil).

This makes a basic soothing balm or salve that can be divided into smaller portions and/or enriched in innumerable ways.

Use herbal infused oils (infused chamomile or calendula) for skin soothing. Add the essential oils of your choice—a drop of peppermint or steam distilled lime for lip balms, lavender and German chamomile for healing baby's diaper rash, and patchouli or frankincense for badly chapped hands. Less beeswax or more of the liquid oil makes a softer balm, more beeswax makes a firm "stick" that can be rubbed on.

basic salt scrub

To 1 cup sea salt, gradually add enough of your favorite rich carrier oil to make a thick paste. (You are aiming for a "wet sand" consistency.) This is a wonderful scrub for calloused feet after a bath or shower. Simply scrub in a small handful of the mix and shower off. Be very careful, this will leave your tub or shower slippery. For an invigorating wakeup, add two drops of peppermint oil. For a relaxing before bedtime spa treatment, add five drops lavender oil.

gentle sugar scrub

If your skin is too sensitive for the Basic Salt Scrub, try this gently exfoliating alternative.

Mix a generous scoop of brown sugar (light or dark will work equally well), enough of your favorite carrier oil to gently moisten, and one or two drops of sandalwood oil. This blend is soothing to the skin, and the aroma is sweetened by the brown sugar. Gently scrub away winter dulled skin, without the sting of salt.

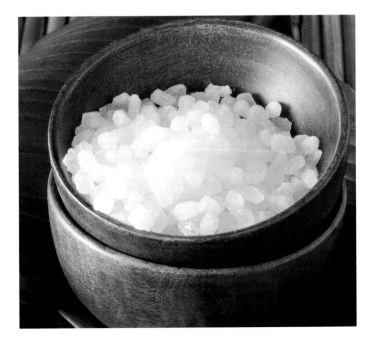

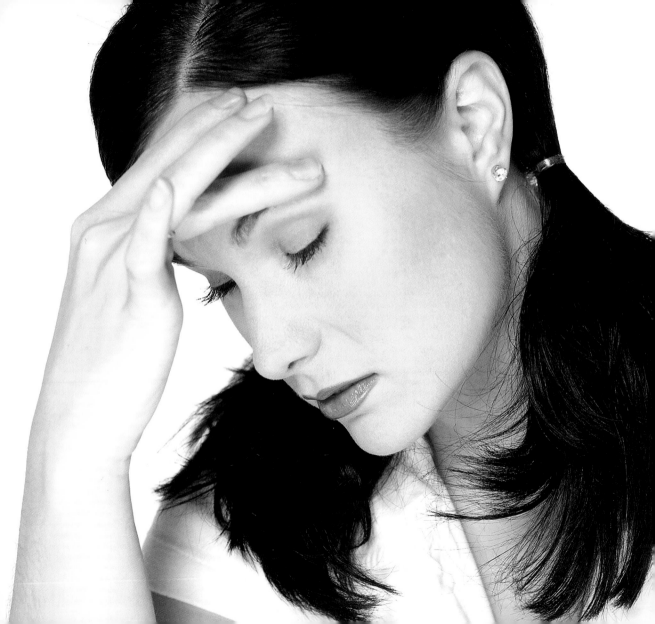

aches and pains

sore muscle blend

4 drops ginger
8 drops rosemary cineole
6 drops Lavandin super
4 drops sweet marjoram

Add 15 drops of the blend to one fluid ounce of carrier oil and massage affected area. Or add 6–8 drops to a blend of Dead Sea salts or Epsom salts and use in a warm bath.

bruise blend

Add 20 drops of Helichrysum italicuum to one ounce of your choice of carrier oil.

sunburn/minor burn blend

10 drops German chamomile
10 drops lavender (I prefer high altitude)
10 drops *Helichrysum Italicuum*

Add 30 drops of the above mixture to 1 fluid ounce jojoba oil. After the essential oils and carrier oil are blended, add 1 fluid ounce aloe vera gel. Shake well. Apply as needed, to ease pain and speed healing.

This is also a powerful soother for insect bites, rashes, and other minor skin irritations.

headache blend

Add 30 drops of lavender or Lavandin super to 1 fluid ounce of carrier oil. Apply to temples and back of neck. Or add 15 drops of peppermint to 1 fluid ounce of carrier oil. Inhale, apply to temples.

sinus congestion/sinus headaches blend

6 drops *Eucalyptus Smithii*
6 drops peppermint
6 drops lavender
3 drops sweet basil

Add 15 drops of the blend to 1 fluid ounce of carrier oil. Apply to sinus areas. Or add 6 drops to a bowl of warm water and inhale. Or just add two drops to a tissue and inhale.

nausea blend

Two essential oils have proven effective at easing nausea, by inhalation. Choose either peppermint essential oil, or ginger essential oil. Put a few drops on a tissue and inhale.

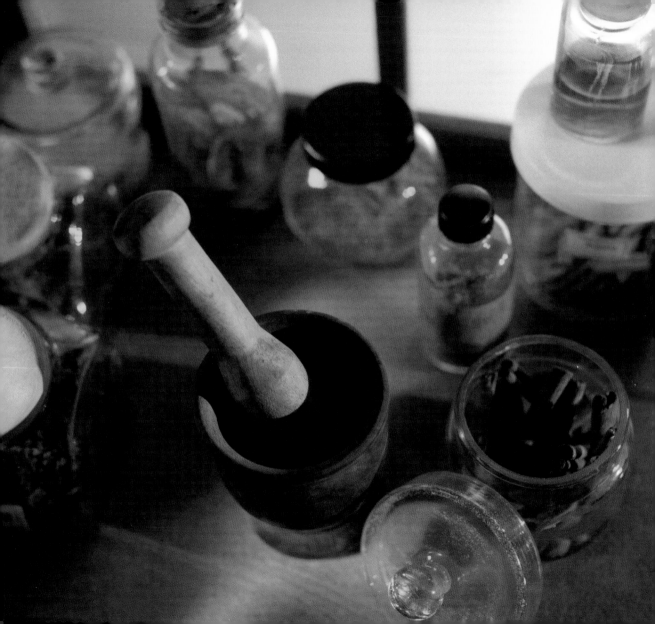

Fragrances for the Home

Essential oils can add vibrance to dull household duties. Certain fragrances can take away nasty smells and some essential oils act as natural and effective cleansers. With these helpful essential oils, you'll find fragrance and function all in one.

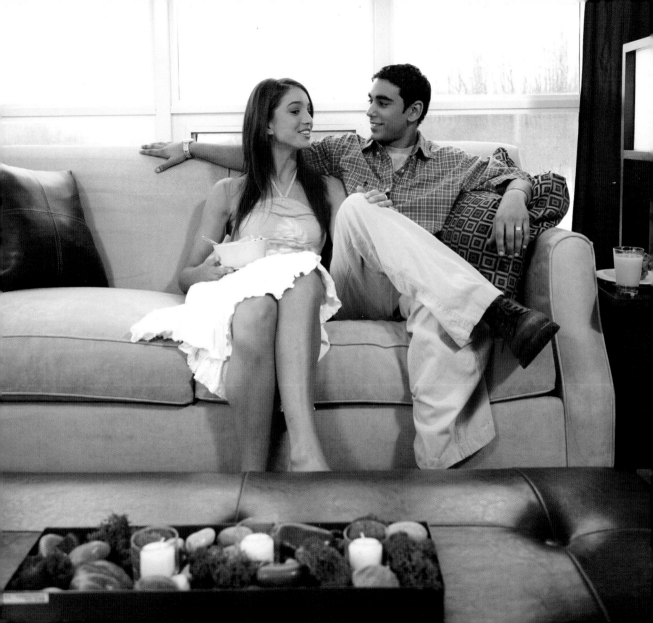

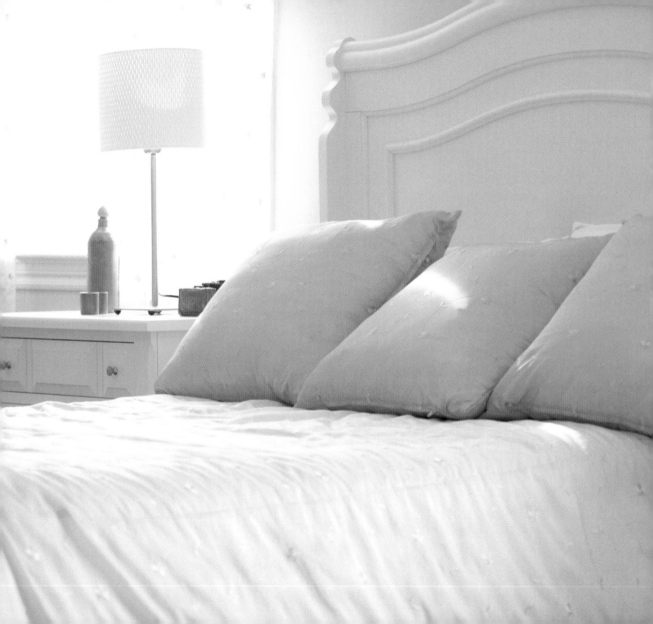

air freshener
10 drops lemon
10 drops bergamot
10 drops lavender

Diffuse to clear smoke and remove cooking or sickroom odors. It works well in the bathroom. This blend is also wonderful in a car. The citrus oils are mood lifters, while the lavender calms irritation, and the car smells fresh and clean. A friend who transported medical patients to and from hospital visits used this blend in his van to keep it clean and fresh smelling.

room freshener
Place in a vaporizer or into a bowl of hot water:
5 drops bergamot
5 drops lemon
5 drops geranium
5 drops clary sage
5 drops basil

This is a good general all-purpose room freshener. A drop or two of just lemon and bergamot will also freshen a room.

bathroom freshener
For the vaporizer:
12 drops lavender or bergamot
2 drops eucalyptus
2 drops juniper

This blend is refreshing and disinfecting.

kitchen freshener

To eliminate cooking smells, add to a vaporizer:

12 drops lemon

12 drops orange

carpet freshener

10 drops *Eucalyptus globulous*

10 drops black spruce

Blend 80 drops of the above (approximately 4 mL or a very scant teaspoonful) into 4 cups of borax (from the laundry detergent aisle of your supermarket). Stir very well to blend the essential oils, and let stand overnight. The next day, sprinkle the mixture over your carpets. Let stand for approximately one hour. Vacuum. Your carpets will be cleaner than they started out, and smell fresh. A great remedy for that "wet dog" odor that those of us who live with a "fur family" can experience.

tennis shoe freshener

20 drops tea tree

10 drops lemon eucalyptus

10 drops Lavandin super

10 drops 'Atlas' cedarwood

Blend together a mixture of 4 tablespoons of baking soda and 4 tablespoons of corn starch. Add 40 drops of the above mixture. Seal tightly, let stand and then sift to blend the essential oils evenly into the dry ingredients.

Add a sprinkle of this to tennis shoes and athletic shoes when they will be able to stand without being worn overnight or for 24 hours. This isn't an "instant" cure-all, but if used regularly you will find a huge improvement in "stinky shoes."

mosquito-/insect repellant

16 drops lemon tea tree
2 drops patchouli
2 drops 'Atlas' cedarwood

Add 15 drops of this blend to either 1 fluid ounce of jojoba or fractionated coconut oil, or one fluid ounce of aloe vera gel.

My experience has been that the oil based blend seems to last longer on the skin. In extreme heat, the aloe based blend tends to be more comfortable.

Note: This is an effective deet-free alternative that has been used by many all over the world.

mold and mildew removal

10 drops tea tree
20 drops lemon eucalyptus

Add approximately 1 teaspoon (5 mL) of this mixture to a bucket of soapy water to loosen and remove mold and mildew. In cases of longstanding problems, I have found that diffusing the blend with a nebulizing diffuser has been extremely helpful.

glass and mirror cleaner

orange essential oil

In a spray bottle, pour 8 ounces (240 mL) of distilled vinegar, add 10 drops of orange oil. Shake well. Add 8 ounces distilled water. Spray, and wipe clean. Orange oil is a wonderful grease cutter, and will leave your house smelling like sunshine.

general germ killer

Use this solution during cold and flu season.

15 drops tea tree
10 drops *Ravensara aromatica*
10 drops lemon oil
5 drops lemon tea tree
5 drops cinnamon leaf

Blend and diffuse to keep bacteria and viruses at bay.

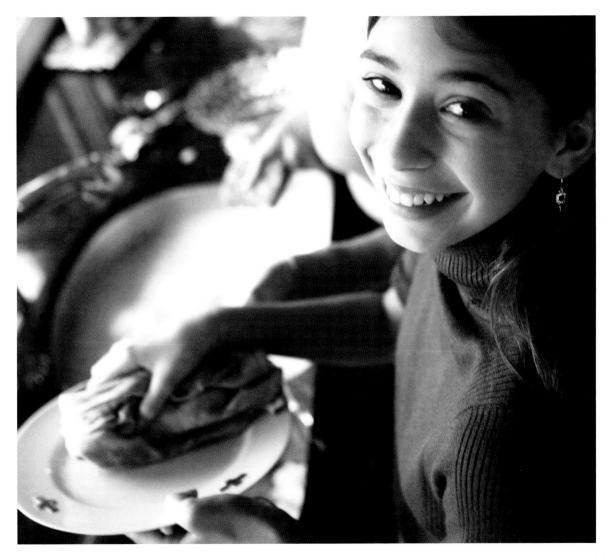

An Alphabetical Guide to the Essential Oils and Their Uses

BASIL, Sweet *Ocimum basilicum*

Basil is considered helpful for mental and physical fatigue, aiding in mental alertness and concentration. A good wake-up oil, used in moderation, a real aid to mental focus and clarity. Helps ease sinus congestion and headaches. Helpful against colds and congestion, as well as easing muscular aches and pains. Avoid use if pregnant or if subject to seizures.

Blends with: citrus oils, black pepper, 'Atlas' cedarwood, clary sage, coriander, cypress, fennel, geranium, ginger, jasmine, juniper, niaouli, palma rosa, pine, rosemary, sage, tea tree, and thyme linalol

BERGAMOT *Citrus bergamia*

Bergamot is an important essential oil for emotional uses. It is encouraging and uplifting, very balancing to the spirit. Bergamot combats fatigue due to stress, tension, and anxiety. It is reputed to strengthen the immune system. Bergamot's aroma is one of the softest and gentlest of the citrus family.

Blends with: It's hard to think of an oil that doesn't blend well with bergamot, but, for a short list: black pepper, clary sage, cypress, frankincense, geranium, *Helichrysum Italicuum*, jasmine, lavender, nutmeg, rosemary, sandalwood, vetiver, and ylang-ylang.

WARNING: Never apply bergamot to skin that will be exposed to the sun. Serious sun damage can result. Bergamot, and some other essential oils, contain substances called furocoumarins which can lead to severe sun poisoning if applied to the skin. There is a "safe" version of bergamot available, steam distilled rather than cold-pressed, with the furocoumarins removed. It will be labeled bergamot FCF, or bergamot Bergaptene-free. Always use this if you are planning an "on the skin" use for this delicate oil.

BLACK PEPPER *Piper nigrum*

Parts used: Dried peppercorns—steam distilled

Black pepper is a mildly stimulating oil. It is wonderful in loosening muscles and relieving the pain of overworked muscles. Aromatically, black pepper is mild and almost woody in aroma. Black pepper oil is a circulatory stimulant. As such, it can be helpful with arthritis, neuralgia, poor circulation, general stiffness, sprains, and sciatica. Emotionally, it is an aphrodisiac and is said to increase self-confidence and to be grounding and stabilizing. Some authorities recommend it for concentration and memory loss. Black pepper is also antibacterial and antiviral, warming and comforting for congestion, the flu, etc. A blend of equal proportions of black pepper, frankincense, jasmine, and sandalwood is absolutely delectable!

Blends with: bergamot, clary sage, clove bud, coriander, fennel, frankincense, geranium, ginger, juniper, lavender, lemongrass, marjoram, myrrh, palma rosa, rosemary, sage, sandalwood, tea tree, vetiver, and ylang-ylang

CARROT SEED *Daucus Carota*

Parts used: Wild carrot seeds—steam distilled

Carrot seed oil is the best essential oil I know for caring for mature skin. It does not have an especially pleasant scent, so I usually blend it with frankincense or neroli, but for skin care products it is unequalled. It is believed to stimulate the red blood cells, adding tone and elasticity to the skin. Carrot seed oil is known for its regenerative powers after severe burns. I include it in my scar treating/reducing blends. For skin care, I prefer to blend it with neroli and perhaps frankincense or *Helichrysum Italicuum*. A base of rose hip seed oil really compliments the anti-aging effect of carrot seed oil.

Blends with: bergamot, juniper berry, lavender, lemon, lime, neroli, orange, petitgrain, and rosemary

CEDARWOOD, Atlas *Cedrus atlantica*

Steam distilled from Morocco, from the wood of relatives of the ancient Cedars of Lebanon.

CEDARWOOD, Himalayan *Cedrus deodora*

Steam distilled from a similar tree that grows high in the Himalayas.

Both 'Atlas' cedarwood and 'Himalayan' cedarwood are excellent for easing the discomfort of any sort of respiratory ailment, either inhaled, or as an ingredient in a "chest rub." They are a must-use for any bronchial congestion. They are often used in treating dandruff and/or oily skin and scalp. Their strong antibacterial action is often recommended for treating bladder and kidney infections, and cystitis (use in a sitz bath or a warm compress applied to the abdomen). Emotionally, cedarwood oil can calm anxiety, and help diffuse fear. It is excellent for insecticide blends. Hang a bit in your closet to keep moths away from your wool clothes. It is an excellent base note for blends containing the "sharper" citrus oils, and nice in a man's blend.

Blends with: all the citrus oils, with vetiver and sandalwood, rose, neroli, rosemary, basil, eucalyptus, and chamomile

CHAMOMILE, German *Matricaria recutita or Matricaria chamomile*

Parts used: Blossoms—steam distilled

German chamomile is a deep cobalt blue essential oil. Colored blue from the chamazulene, a soothing component that makes German chamomile a wonderful choice for treating inflamed, irritated skin. Dilute in carrier oil or use in a compress for any sort of inflammation. German chamomile excels at treating all sorts of dry, itchy flaky skin problems. This deep blue oil is most effective used in carrier oil and applied to the skin. I see very little use for it in a diffuser or lamp. I know of nothing better to add to a blend for treating infected skin and acne, or to blend with lavender for sunburn than this. I put it in my grand baby's baby oil, along with lavender to treat the occasional touch of diaper rash. German chamomile oil is recommended for treating any sort of rash or skin irritation. A must for treating rosacea and/or couperose, an essential ingredient in our anti-acne blend, also you might blend with lavender for treating sun and windburn.

Blends with: bergamot, jasmine, labdanum, lavender, neroli, clary sage, and rose

CHAMOMILE, Roman *Anthemis Nobilis*

Parts used: Flower—steam distilled

Roman chamomile is much sweeter smelling than German. It smells the way chamomile tea tastes, and is the only steam distilled chamomile I have found that does. I prefer to use Roman chamomile for inhalation, as a sedative or pain reliever. Roman chamomile is wonderful for insomnia caused by stress or tension and for relieving intestinal spasms (especially when blended with sweet marjoram). It is helpful for inflamed joints and muscle or joint pain. It's a wonderfully calming pain and stress reliever. Useful to combat pain of arthritis and/or menstrual cramps, as well as insomnia and headaches. I tend to use the German chamomile for skin disorders, and the Roman for internal "aches and pains." The Roman is better for relaxing and summoning sleep. Try rubbing a bit of Roman chamomile on the back of the neck and the temples before visiting the dentist. I've read that this can ease anxiety as well as support the action of the anesthetic used.

Blends with: cinnamon, bergamot, clary sage, geranium, jasmine, cistus, neroli, lemon, lavender, sweet marjoram, orange, rose, rosewood, sandalwood, ylang-ylang, and oakmoss.

CINNAMON LEAF *Cinnamomum zeylanicum*

Please note, we do not recommend cinnamon bark essential oil for beginner's use. It is both a strong skin irritant and a sensitizer. Not safe in any dilution for skin use. Cinnamon leaf, on the other hand, may be used with caution in very low dilutions. We still recommend limiting its use to the aroma lamp or room sprays. Cinnamon leaf oil is far less sensitizing than cinnamon bark oil, but it is still a skin irritant and possible sensitizer so it should be used highly diluted. Cinnamon leaf is a powerful broad spectrum anti-infectious and antifungal. It can be an effective addition to tooth and gum care blends. Some authorities recommend it for feelings of isolation, loneliness, and fear.

Blends with: black pepper, caraway, citrus oils, clove bud, eucalyptus, frankincense, ginger, grapefruit, lavender, lemon, myrtle, nutmeg, orange, rosemary, thyme, and tea tree

WARNING: Cinnamon leaf is a strong skin irritant. Please avoid use during pregnancy or with children under five. Cinnamon leaf may induce menstruation or stimulate childbirth contractions. Avoid use of cinnamon leaf if you are on anti-coagulant therapy (blood thinners).

CLARY SAGE *Salvia sclarea*

Parts used: Flowering tops—steam distilled

Clary sage is a necessary oil for every woman. It helps ease menstrual cramps, balances PMS, and eases the pangs of menopause. Add clary sage's hormonal properties to geranium for almost any sort of "female problems," both physical and emotional. For skin care, clary sage can help inhibit excessive perspiration, and may be useful in treating very greasy scalp conditions. Clary can help balance extreme emotions, reducing stress and restoring inner tranquility. Equal amounts of clary sage, lavender, and ylang-ylang make a wonderfully feminine stress relieving diffuser or aroma lamp blend.

Blends with: bergamot, 'Atlas' cedarwood, all chamomiles, frankincense, geranium, jasmine, lavender, sweet marjoram, neroli, orange, rosewood, sandalwood, and ylang-ylang

WARNING: Avoid using clary while drinking alcohol, and avoid while pregnant or nursing. It is also contraindicated in cases of estrogen-dependant cancers.

CLOVE *Eugenia carophyllata*

Parts used: Dried flower bud—steam distilled

Clove has one valuable first aid benefit—it numbs the nerves. This quality makes it a valuable emergency treatment for a toothache. Just a drop of diluted clove oil on a cotton swab applied to the sore tooth—not to the surrounding gum area—can provide dramatic relief from the pain of a toothache. Clove is also stimulating to the mind and memory, helpful in cases of fatigue and/or depression. Clove is an essential oil to be used with caution and respect.

WARNING: Clove oil is a known dermal and mucous membrane irritant and sensitizer. It should not be used on the skin, or, if necessary, used in very weak dilution (less than 1%). It should not ever be applied to broken or irritated skin. Avoid use of any clove oil if you are on anti-coagulant therapy (blood thinners).

EUCALYPTUS SPECIES

The most commonly known eucalyptus oil is *Eucalyptus globulous* but there are several different varieties of eucalyptus with varying effects and uses.

BLUE GUM EUCALYPTUS
Eucalyptus globulous

Parts used: Leaves—steam distilled

Eucalyptus is best known for its respiratory effects. It fights viruses and bacteria, while easing congestion. It also eases muscle and joint aches and pains. *Eucalyptus globulous* stimulates circulation, increasing the flow of blood to affected areas. Eucalyptus can be mentally stimulating and may help increase concentration. As far as blending goes, eucalyptus is going to dominate any blend it's used in, so it should be blended with essentials that contribute to the effect you want to achieve. Frankincense compliments its respiratory effects. Bergamot, blended with eucalyptus, can reduce the discomfort of cold sores, herpes outbreaks, and shingles. The combination is reputed to be effective against that specific virus.

Blends with: basil, cajeput, cedarwood, cypress, lavender, lemon, rosemary, and pine

WARNING: Do not use with infants and small children; it can cause choking.

LEMON EUCALYPTUS *Eucalyptus Citriodora*

Parts used: Leaves—steam distilled

Light, lemony, and refreshing, this eucalyptus is a wonderful air freshener. It appears to have anti-staph effects. It is a strong antifungal oil, and we have used it in the diffuser after a flood that soaked the carpeting with groundwater. *Eucalyptus citriodora* did a superb job of removing the musty smell left over. It is also often recommended as an insect repellant. Lemon eucalyptus can be very sedating in small quantities.

Blends with: cedarwood and patchouli

EUCALYPTUS RADIATA *Eucalyptus radiata*

Parts used: Leaves—steam distilled

My friend says this is the most useful eucalyptus because it smells better and is more easily assimilated. It is most useful for sinus conditions because it can be inhaled closely without triggering a cough reflex. Many sources say it is the oil of choice for infections high up in the chest.

EUCALYPTUS SMITHII *Eucalyptus smithii*

Parts used: Leaves—steam distilled

This is the mildest of the eucalyptus, safe for children and the elderly. It is recommend as a preventative as it affects the entire respiratory system and immune system. *Eucalyptus smithii* makes a good room disinfector in a diffuser, but can trigger a cough reflex if breathed too close. It is one of the best oils for painful joints and muscles.

FRANKINCENSE *Boswellia carterii*

Parts used: Resin—steam distilled or CO_2-extracted

Frankincense has traditionally been used for spiritual growth and meditation. It is believed to have a centering effect on the emotions. It can slow respiration, thus helping your body calm and center itself. Frankincense can act as an expectorant, soothing congestion while also relaxing breathing. In skin care, frankincense is a wonderful oil to blend into facial creams or oils for aging skin. Frankincense tends to "soften" any sharply scented oil blended with it and seems to blend well with any of the woods or spices.

Blends with: grapefruit, orange, lemon, lavender, sandalwood, patchouli, rose, and vetiver

GERANIUM or ROSE GERANIUM
Pelargonium graveolens or Pelargonium roseum

Parts used: Leaves—steam distilled

Geranium's aroma is softly floral as well as green. A "woman's oil," geranium seems to have a hormonal balancing effect and traditionally has been used (blended with clary sage) to alleviate problems associated with menopause and menstruation. It also acts as a diuretic. It can lower blood sugar and should be avoided if you are hypoglycemic. Geranium and rose geranium are valuable skin care oils. They are helpful for bruises, cuts, ulcers, broken capillaries, dermatitis, and as anti-inflammatories. It is believed to balance sebum (making it the oil of choice for combination skin) and to keep the skin smooth and supple. The only oils I don't like in combination with it are the citrus oils. They seem to "sharpen" it too much for my taste.

Blends with: clary sage, rose, sandalwood, frankincense, lavender, and chamomile

GINGER *Zingiber officinale*

Parts used: Roots—steam distilled (Ginger oil is available distilled from both fresh and dried roots. The fresh root yields a much more aromatically pleasing essential oil.)

Ginger is one of my favorite oils. The steam-distilled specimen is a skin irritant and needs using with a light hand, but should be safe for the skin in normal aromatherapy dilutions. Ginger oil, for those who have not tried it, is wonderfully soothing for aching joints and muscles, or an upset stomach. Ginger's heat can be irritating to the skin, so be sure to dilute it. It is a wonderful ingredient in massage blends for aching muscles or as a warming ingredient in a "chest rub" for a cold or flu. Recent studies have indicated that cinnamon leaf and ginger, in synergy, are an effective analgesic and rubifactant. The combination of the two are more effective at lower dilutions than either one alone. Ginger can be an aphrodisiac and has been used by some to treat male impotence. Ginger blends well with the citrus oils, and the woods or resins. To ease an upset stomach or heartburn, we usually add one drop of ginger oil, mixed into a teaspoon of honey in a cup. Fill with hot water, stir, and drink. Instant ginger tea!

Blends with: black pepper, fennel, lemongrass, all citrus oils, all wood oils, most resins, lavender and eucalyptus (for pain relief)

GRAPEFRUIT *Citrus paradisii*

Parts used: Rind—cold pressed

I never particularly liked grapefruit essential oil until I discovered pink grapefruit. It fairly sparkles, it's so bright and crisp, both energizing and uplifting. Grapefruit is recommended by some authorities for treating eating disorders, both anorexia and overeating, when they stem from lack of self-esteem. Of all the citrus oils, pink grapefruit is by far the most energizing. Physically, pink grapefruit oil is helpful in treating oily skin and hair. Pink grapefruit, applied topically, is recommended as part of anti-cellulite blends because of its toning and astringent

effects. It has been shown to stimulate the lymphatic system, and thus help the body remove toxins.

Blends with: all conifers (especially cypress and juniper), other citrus oils, and eucalyptus

HELICHRYSUM, Italian Everlasting
Helichrysum Italicum

Parts used: Blossoms—steam distilled

There are many varieties of helichrysum essential oil commercially available. The only helichrysum you should purchase is *Helichrysum Italicum*, grown and distilled on the island of Corsica, off the coast of France. Others are less costly than this rare specimen, but will not give you the healing results.

The steam-distilled oil of the Italian Everlasting is one of the strongest anti-inflammatories I know. I use it in all my skin blends. The fragrance is warm, slightly honey-like, rich and buttery, with green notes of wood, spices, and herbs. It is a fascinating oil because it is made up of several layers of notes that appear to unfold during the dry down. *Helichrysum Italicuum* is antibacterial, antiviral, and antifungal. A strong dilution of *Helichrysum Italicuum* in a base of rose hip seed carrier oil has shown amazing results in healing/fading surgical scars and scars left from burns. Any blend created for arthritis, bruising, or scarring needs *Helichrysum Italicuum*. We have seen amazing relief from arthritis pain and various joint pains from using a blend of *Helichrysum Italicuum*, black pepper, and lavender oil in a base of anti-inflammatory St. John's Wort infused oil. Mentally and emotionally, *Helichrysum Italicuum* is very supportive and comforting. It is believed by some to open the right side of the brain and improve creativity as well as increase dream activity. In my experience, it is the most healing of all essential oils.

Blends with: boronia, chamomile, all citrus oils, clary sage, clove, cypress, geranium, lavender, mimosa, neroli, oakmoss, patchouli, rose, and vetiver

JASMINE ABSOLUTE

Parts used: Blossoms—solvent extracted

As rose is traditionally known as the queen of flowers, jasmine is the king. It is essential for anyone with an interest in perfumery, but offers much more than just a lovely exotic aroma. Jasmine is often recommended for use during childbirth. It is said to strengthen contractions, relieve pain, and aid post-natal recovery. It is also recommended by some as a hormone balancer or a soother for menstrual pain. It is often used in skin care, especially in the treatment of dry or aggravated skin. Many use it in treating eczema and dermatitis, however it can be sensitizing and I'd not recommend using it on problem skin. It is in its emotional uses that jasmine truly shines. Almost every authority recommends it as an aphrodisiac,

especially for those who lack confidence in their own sexuality. It is said to be as powerful an antidepressant as ylang-ylang, basil, and melissa.

Blends with: bergamot, clary, frankincense, geranium, lavender, orange, mandarin, neroli, palma rosa, rose, rosewood, sandalwood, and ylang-ylang

There are three available species of jasmine Absolutes:

JASMINE GRANDIFLORA
Jasminun grandiflorum

'Jasmine Grandiflora' is much more widely known than the other varieties described below. It is the jasmine grown in Europe and Northern Africa, and usually the specimen grown in the U.S. The 'Grandiflora' is much more commonly used in perfumery than its rarer cousin. Jasmine 'Grandiflora's' aroma is softer, more gentle, and less exotic than that of the 'Sambac'. As the 'Sambac' blossoms seem to capture the mystery of the night and the moonlight, the dawn-blooming 'Grandiflora' seems to carry the essence of a bright new day.

JASMINE SAMBAC
Jasminun officianalis sambac

To my nose, this is the jasmine with the richest, most heady aroma. If you are looking for an exotic scent, this is your choice! The opening notes of 'Jasmine Sambac' are heavy and sweet with a richness and mysterious depth. As the scent develops, there are both fruity and floral notes. The 'Grandiflora' is softer, more feminine; while the 'Sambac' truly deserves the name "the King of Flowers."

Note: 8,000 individual blossoms (carefully hand-picked) are required to produce 1 gram—approximately 1 mL—of absolute. No bruised flowers may be used for extraction, since their aroma is ruined by bruising or mishandling.

JASMINE AURICULATUM
Jasminun auriculatus

This much less known jasmine is a total delight. The experts describe it as having a rich, gardenia-like aroma. It is intensely floral, but with a rich rounded fruity aroma, underlying the radiant floral notes. Even those of us who normally find our other jasmine species a bit too lush for our taste fell in love with this.

JUNIPER BRANCH with BERRY or JUNIPER BERRY
Juniperus communis

Parts used: Branch tips with berries—steam distilled

Juniper is said to clean the atmosphere of a room and assist with meditation.

Physically, it is a diuretic and is often included in anti-cellulite and detoxifying blends. (Try blending with grapefruit and fennel for cellulite.) It is an essential component of any detoxifying blend. Juniper oil is said to help in recovering from hangovers. It may be helpful with arthritis and rheumatism. Do not use during pregnancy. I personally like it blended with a touch of lemon, sandalwood, cypress, or frankincense. It is a key ingredient in all detoxifying synergies and baths. Avoid with kidney disease and acute bladder/kidney infections.

Blends with: cypress, eucalyptus, grapefruit, lemon, fennel, frankincense, and rosemary

LAVENDER

Parts used: Flowering tops—steam distilled

All lavender oils are not alike. There are three commonly available Lavandula species oils: 'True' lavender (*Lavandula angustifolia* or *Lavandula officianalis*), 'Spike' lavender (*Lavandula spica* or *Lavandula latifolia*) and lavandin (*Lavandula hybrid var xxx*).

TRUE LAVENDER
Lavandula angustifolia or *Lavandula officianalis*

Parts used: Flowering tops—steam distilled

Lavender is often known as the "all-purpose" essential oil, and the starting point of most people's aromatic journey. Lavender oil is antibacterial, antifungal, and perhaps antiviral. It is an anti-inflammatory for skin care, and is useful for all skin types, especially useful in treating acne and rosacea. It can be a pain reliever, and a necessary component of sore muscle blends. A few drops of lavender in the bath can ease tension and help prevent insomnia. In very weak dilutions, it can help soothe baby's diaper rash. In fact, it is the first essential oil recommended for use with babies.

Lavender essential oil is a virtual "first aid" cabinet in and of itself. A touch of lavender essential oil on the temples and back of the neck can ease a headache. A drop of lavender can soothe and help heal a minor burn. A compress with lavender oil can help the pain and infection of a boil; can ease the pain of a sprained or strained muscle. Lavender is lovely in the bath. A lavender bath will relax tired muscles and a tired mind. It's a wonderful way to relax before bedtime.

Ten to fifteen drops of lavender mixed into an ounce of your favorite carrier oil makes a wonderfully relaxing massage oil.

Try to sample the lavender essential oil you are buying before purchasing. Lavender originating from different countries will have very different aromas. The finest lavender commercially available is probably French high altitude lavender grown from seed, sometimes labeled lavender fine or lavender population. Distilling at higher altitudes allows more of the delicate aromatic esters to come across during distillation, creating a higher quality essential oil. High altitude lavender oil should have a crisp cleanly floral aroma. Growing from seed—not cloning the plants—gives a different energy to the plant and its oil. It feels more vibrant and alive. My favorite lavender, aromatically, is a French clone, called 'Mailette'. The growers clone the plants to achieve more consistency in the yield from one harvest to another, and to breed in the qualities they want. It has the most delightful velvety aroma. The 'Mailette' is particularly high in linalyl acetate, which gives it an extra sweetness. A truly delightful oil. Bulgarian lavender, to my nose, has a slightly less clear and distinctive aroma, but is unsurpassed as a sedative. It is the lavender that I reach for when insomnia is stalking my nights. Lavender grown and distilled high in the Himalayan mountains in India and Nepal has a delightfully crisp almost "green" scent. I find it blends better with the citrus oils than other lavenders do. It seems a bit less relaxing than the European lavenders, so it is not my choice for evening use, but is a wonderful addition to air freshening sprays. The lavender oil that I have sampled from Africa seems much more camphorous than the European grown. I suspect it would make an excellent antibacterial, but to my nose it is less pleasing than other specimens of true lavender.

Blends with: (almost everything!) Aromatically, lavender blends beautifully with geranium and rose geranium, and clary sage. It compliments rose, and the oils that have "rosy" aromas, such as rosewood and palma rosa. It blends well with most other floral and herbal oils. For pain relief, add one of the warming spice oils, ginger or black pepper, or eucalyptus oil. To heighten its antibacterial effects, blend with tea tree. For irritated skin, blend with German chamomile or *Helichrysum Italicuum*. To soothe a fretful toddler, try blending with Roman chamomile or mandarin, tangerine, or sweet orange. To help lower a fever, sponge the body or use a cool compress of peppermint and lavender. There truly is no end to the oils that lavender will blend with, and to its uses.

SPIKE LAVENDER
Lavandula spica or lavandula latifolia

Parts used: Flowering tops—steam distilled

Now, 'Spike' is not at all your "usual" lavender. This one is not recommended for infants, children, or the elderly. 'Spike' lavender is higher in cineole and camphor, which makes it an effective addition to respiratory blends, and useful for general aches and pains. It is also a very potent germ killer. Some authorities recommend spike as an insect repellant, and say it is useful for hair and skin care. It would be a good addition to anti-acne blends, but I would avoid using it for sensitive skin. A stimulant, rather than a sedative, do not use for relaxation.

Blends with: peppermint, tea tree, rosemary, eucalyptus, and cedarwood

WARNING: Avoid use with anyone with a seizure disorder, with children, with the elderly or frail.

LAVANDIN *Lavandula hybrid*

Lavandin is not true lavender. It is the result of a cross between lavender vera and 'Spike' lavender, sometimes known as aspic. True lavender grows higher in the mountains, while 'Spike' lavender is a lowland plant. Originally, at the borders of their geographic territory, the seeds mixed and wild lavandin began to grow. No hybrid will set seeds, so all the lavandin oil commercially available is a result of clones of the original plants.

There are several varieties of lavandin available, each with a different aroma, and different therapeutic properties.

Lavandula hybrid var. super

Lavandin super is the lavandin closest to true lavender aromatically, and, since it produces much more essential oil than *Lavandula angustifolia*, is often used to extend or adulterate true lavender oil. Like true lavender, it is a soothing, relaxing oil when used in moderation. Antispasmodic and relaxing, it is the gentlest of the lavandins. It is a wonderful oil to use in a relaxing bath or massage. My Belgian friend uses two drops taken internally as his recommended migraine remedy. (Please don't take any essential oil internally unless you are under the direct care of a trained aromatherapist!)

I would strongly recommend this lavandin for treating headaches—migraine, and otherwise.

Lavandula hybrid var. grosso

Lavandin grosso is less floral than the 'Super' described above. It has a touch of spice to its aroma, mixed with the herbal lavender notes. *Lavandin grosso* produces far more essential oil than the other lavandins, which in turn produce a great deal more essential oil than do the true lavenders. Of today's French production, 90% is *Lavandin grosso*. It and the other lavandins are often used to adulterate true lavender. I find the 'Super' a bit more relaxing and still prefer it for relaxation and stress relief, but for inflammation, the *Lavandin grosso* definitely has a role to play. It is a good antiseptic and stimulating oil and is useful in treating skin conditions such as acne and sluggish skin. I've seen it recommended as the oil of choice for scabies and other infectious skin diseases. It is a good addition to cold and flu remedies with its proven germ-killing ability, as well as its ability to stimulate the respiratory system and ease breathing. A blend of *Lavandin grosso* and 'Spike' lavender is recommended for respiratory disorders, either by inhalation or massage.

Lavandula hybrid var. abrialis

A bit of lavender history is still alive in this lovely specimen. *Lavandin abrial* was the first successfully cloned lavandin. Lavandin abrial oil is high in linalyl acetate, one of the benchmark components of fine *Lavender angustifolia*. (High altitude lavender contains much more linalyl acetate than does its lowland cousins, and aromatically this *Lavandin abrial* is closer to high altitude than to French 'Mailette.') *Lavandin abrial* is an effective mucolytic and expectorant. It is much gentler than 'Spike' lavender, which has the similar effects, and thus more appropriate for diffusion with children. *Lavandin abrial* specific components make it a wonderful "support oil" to be used with the various eucalyptus oils, tea tree, and manuka.

LEMON OIL *Citrus limon*

Parts used: Rind or zest—cold pressed (It is also available steam distilled, but the aroma is disappointing.)

Tart, tangy true lemon aroma, smelling just like fresh grated lemon zest. Lemon oil is a strong germicide and astringent, a wonderful air disinfectant and freshener. I use it in cleaning solutions all the time for its clean scent and disinfecting action. Lemon essential oil has fever reducing action as well as effective germicidal action, so it's a good oil to use to aid in treating colds and fevers.

Lemon oil stimulates the immune system and circulation. Lemon is a key component in most anti-cellulite blends. It has a toning effect on oily skin and hair. Lemon oil also has powerful effects on the mind. It refreshes and rejuvenates. It is an aid to mental focus and alertness. Lemon is a wonderful oil to diffuse in a car, to help the driver stay alert, or in a "study blend" or any blend that intends to improve mental focus.

Of all the oils where organic as opposed to conventional farming methods make a difference, the citrus fruit oils lead the way. After all, when a crop is sprayed with insecticides, it is the rind of the lemon that is coated with and absorbs the chemicals. Research has shown appallingly high levels of pesticides in many essential oils. The use of organic cold pressed oils will eliminate the chemical residue completely.

Blends with: 'Atlas' cedarwood, lavender, neroli, patchouli, peppermint, any of the coniferous oils, many of the spice oils, and other citrus oils

LEMONGRASS *Cymbopogon flexuosus*

Parts used: Grass leaves—steam distilled

Historically, the herbal form of lemongrass has been used in traditional Indian medicine for infectious illnesses and fever. The essential oil is stimulating and invigorating. It is helpful for treating symptoms of jet lag, clearing the head, and relieving fatigue. Lemongrass essential oil is considered an excellent physical tonic. It is said to boost the parasympathetic nervous system, which hastens recovery from illness. Lemongrass is an effective skin toner, said to be effective for tightening open pores. There are

those who recommend it for treating acne and oily skin. I do not recommend using it on troubled skin since it can be a skin irritant.

MANDARIN

Parts used: Rind—cold pressed

With all of these cold pressed citrus rind oils I would urge you to seek out organically grown oils. When the citrus fields are sprayed with pesticides, they cover the rind and are then carried into the essential oil.

All of these citrus subspecies—green mandarin, red mandarin, clementine, and tangerine—are gentle, mild, and emotionally uplifting. Their primary use is in the aroma lamp or diffuser. I call them the "citrus smile bringers." Gentle enough to use with toddlers, they are the most delightful mood altering substances that I know of. Many authorities say they can be used interchangeably, however there are definite aromatic differences among them, and each has its own special purpose. However, if a formula calls for one, and you have another, feel free to substitute. Please remember that all cold pressed citrus oils have the potential to cause photosensitization (sun damage) and should not be applied to the skin within 12 hours of exposure to sunlight or ultraviolet light.

All blend well with bergamot, neroli, rose, sandalwood, and ylang-ylang.

GREEN MANDARIN *citrus deliciosa*

Clear green in color, and deliciously tart in fragrance, green mandarin is like no citrus oil I've experienced. Perhaps a blend of lime, lemon, orange, and key lime? It is tart, energizing, and uplifting. A delightful morning oil.

RED MANDARIN *citrus nobilis*

Similar in uses to tangerine, but much more complex and adult in aroma, mandarin is gentle enough to use with young children and during pregnancy. Red mandarin tends to be more tart than tangerine or green mandarin, and more complex, aromatically. It is a great antiseptic to use as a room spray and a toner for oily or blemished skin. But where mandarin really shines is in its emotional uses. It is considered both a calming influence and gently uplifting. Wonderful for use with children, a true "citrus smile bringer." Mandarin is also a wonderful treatment for sleep disturbances and insomnia.

WARNING: Mildly phototoxic, do not apply before going out in the sun.

CLEMENTINE *Citrus reticulata*

Parts used: Rind—cold pressed

Over a decade ago, I fell in love with clementine oil. It is as complex and multi-layered as a good red mandarin, but sweeter. It has the sweetness of sweet orange rind or tangerine, but more subtle. There's almost a touch of floral to it. I love this deep reddish orange oil. It is another species of tangerine, for those who have never experienced it, so it is gentle and safe enough to use with toddlers. A mild photosensitizer, and like all citrus oils, mildly irritating to the skin, so I would be very cautious on the skin use. But, ah, for the aroma lamp or diffuser, it is a joy. Relaxing, not energizing, clementine oil fills the room with calm, quiet, and peace.

TANGERINE *Citrus reticulata var Dancy*

Parts used: Rind—cold pressed

This is the younger cousin of my favorite mandarin oil, softer, sweeter, lacking the complexity of mandarin, but a perfect child's oil with its sweetness. Tangerine is a delightful alternative to orange oil, a bit lighter and much sweeter when used in a blend. Emotionally, it is cheering and strengthening. Pregnant women and young children seem to enjoy it. I use it in a room spray or the aroma lamp with a touch of basil to keep me "up."

Many authors say tangerine and mandarin may be used interchangeably, but I find their scents very different. Red mandarin seems a bit tarter, closer to a blend of orange and grapefruit, and much more complex. Tangerine is wonderfully sweet, a true "citrus smile bringer." Tangerine is a wonderful oil to diffuse in a toddler's room, or to add to his bath. As with all the citrus oils, beware of photosensitivity.

MARJORAM, Sweet *Origanum marjorana*

Parts used: Flowers and leaves—steam distilled

Marjoram's aroma is slightly spicy, warm, and soothing. Marjoram has been used to lower high blood pressure. It warms the skin, where applied. Marjoram's powerful antispasmodic action can ease pains of arthritis, cramped muscles, muscle spasms, and menstrual cramps. (Try blending with clary sage for relieving menstrual cramps; the result is almost magical!) It has a calming, slightly sedative action and can be effective against some types of migraines. I sometimes blend it with clary sage, especially for menstrual difficulties. Sweet marjoram mixes well with lavender or rosewood or 'English' chamomile for a very relaxing bath.

Blends with: orange, geranium, eucalyptus (softening it, somewhat) and lavender

WARNING: Marjoram can stimulate menstrual flow, and thus should never be used during pregnancy.

MELISSA *Melissa officianalis*

Parts used: Leaves—steam distilled

Probably the most rare herbal essential oil is that distilled from the common lemon balm. Almost all so-called melissa oil on the commercial market is a mixture of lemongrass and citronella. True melissa is expensive because, although the plant is easy to grow, it takes approximately three tons of plant material to yield 1 pound (.5kg) of the essential oil.

This light, clear lemony oil is a delight to the senses and the emotions. Its aroma is clear, clean, and icy-cool, not medicinal or citronella murky. Medicinally, melissa essential oil has been confirmed to have powerful antiviral properties. Said to be useful against various strains of flu virus, herpes, smallpox, and mumps. Melissa is also recommended for treatment of both nausea and indigestion, especially when they are caused by nervous tension. Some authorities say that it slows the heartbeat, relieving palpitations, and helps lower blood pressure. Blended with geranium, it may help ease painful periods.

Emotionally, melissa is a delight. It is a mild sedative in small doses, and believed to calm anxiety. Both calming and uplifting, melissa essential oil is said to be extremely useful in cases of emotional shock, grief, fear, and anger. It is said to bring acceptance and understanding.

WARNING: Melissa essential oil is a strong skin irritant, and needs to be used in very low dilutions. I would limit it to approximately five drops per ounce of carrier, or two to three drops in a bath.

MYRRH *Commiphora myrrha*

Parts used: Resin—hydro distilled

Myrrh, another of the ancient "sacred oils" has been used as an astringent for thousands of years. Myrrh is an effective antifungal and antibacterial oil. It clears extra mucous from the lungs and is useful for helping "dry out" respiratory problems. It can help ease the itching and irritation of weeping eczema, and helps fight the fungus that causes jock strap itch. Its most popular and effective use is in treating gum diseases and sores in the mouth. It makes an excellent mouthwash to promote oral health. It is said to stimulate menstrual flow, and thus should be avoided during pregnancy.

Blends with: frankincense (of course, for meditation blends), rose or patchouli (for skin care), and peppermint (for oral use)

NEROLI *Citrus aurantium var. amara*

Parts used: Blossoms—steam distilled

The bitter orange tree gives us three very different essential oils: bitter orange, cold pressed from the rind of the fruit, petitgrain, steam distilled from the leaves and immature fruit, and true neroli, distilled from the blossoms. Much of the so-called neroli on the market is a distillation of blossoms and leaves together. It is much less expensive to produce, but aromatically quite different from the true, blossom-only neroli. This is oil that you truly must sample from several sources so that your nose will recognize the green, leaf-note of the oil that comes from leaves mixed in with the flowers. Once you have experienced true, blossom-only neroli, you will never again be fooled by the lower quality.

Neroli's aroma is a wonderful blend of floral with undertones of citrus. Emotionally, neroli can help calm anxiety and relieve depression. It is a key ingredient in any anti-anxiety blend. I have seen a drop of pure neroli oil bring a panic attack to a smooth, calm halt. Neroli can help balance both oily and dry skin, since it has a sebum balancing effect. It is a wonderful skin care oil for mature skin, as well. There is also an orange blossom absolute, solvent extracted from the same blossoms that give us neroli essential oil. Aromatically, it is closer to the scent of the fresh blossoms, but it lacks the therapeutic and skin care properties of the steam distilled oil. It is produced for perfumery, not aromatherapy.

Blends with: bergamot, frankincense, sandalwood, petitgrain, rose, lemon, orange, lavender, patchouli, and vetiver

ORANGE, Sweet *Citrus sinensis*

Parts used: Peel—cold pressed (There is a steam distilled orange rind oil, and an oil distilled from the fruit itself, but both are aromatically inferior.)

The essential oil of the sweet orange is delightfully bright and cheery and is a strong antidepressant. Used in the aroma lamp, it brightens the atmosphere of a room. Blended with any of the spice or coniferous oils, it makes a wonderful winter holiday blend. Orange is refreshing and relaxing. It can cause photosensitivity, so be careful of applying to the skin prior to exposure to sunlight. It is generally considered mild enough for use with small children.

As said earlier, of all the oils where organic as opposed to conventional farming methods make a difference, the citrus fruit oils lead the way. After all, when a crop is sprayed with insecticides, it is the rind of the orange that is coated with and absorbs the chemicals. Many of these chemicals carry through to the essential oils, and more are contained in cold pressed oils. The use of organic cold pressed oils will eliminate the chemical residue completely. If you love orange, you owe it to yourself to try this.

Blends with: bergamot, geranium, lavender, neroli, petitgrain, rosewood, sandalwood, ylang-ylang, and all woods and spices

PATCHOULI *Pogostemon patchouli*

Parts used: Grass—steam distilled

Patchouli, oil of the '60s, is an effective anti-inflammatory for the skin, helpful in healing cracked or inflamed skin, acne, dermatitis, and eczema. It is said to tone and tighten the skin, and is used in many anti-wrinkle blends. At the same time, it helps regulate oily skin and dandruff. Some authorities say it is useful in appetite suppressant blends and, with its skin-toning qualities, in combating cellulite.

It is an excellent base note for perfume blends, and is generally considered an aphrodisiac. In small quantities, it has a mildly sedative effect, while in large quantities, it may be stimulating.

Please keep in mind that patchouli is very thick and may have a hard time coming out of the orifice reducers in the bottles. You'll most likely need to take the orifice reducer out and pipette the patchouli out. Be sure to replace the orifice reducer, as it is what creates a seal between the bottle and top.

Blends with: all citrus oils, all woods, rose, neroli, and most spice oils

Patchouli is a very intense oil and while wonderful for "anchoring" a blend, making it last longer on the skin, it needs to be blended with a very light hand. It can easily overpower the more delicate "top notes" in a blend.

PEPPERMINT *Mentha x Piperita*

Peppermint essential oil is one of the "basic necessities" for a first aid kit. It is one of the oils often recommended for easing migraines (especially those stemming from digestive problems); it helps clear congestion in the sinuses. It can ease indigestion—just add one drop on a sugar cube, or in a spoonful of honey.

Mentally, it clears the brain, helps concentration, is a restorative in cases of mental fatigue, and acts as a mental stimulant. Peppermint is not an oil to use in the evening when you are seeking sleep, but is great in the car to help keep the driver alert. Peppermint is the ideal remedy for all digestive disorders, including nausea and vomiting. It is a great remedy for car or air sickness. In a massage, it helps stimulate the lymph system. It is also an analgesic and aids with treating sore muscles and joint pain. In skin care, a very weak dilution (less than 1%) is helpful for easing itching or irritation. We add a few drops to calamine lotion to treat poison ivy. Definitely a case where "less is more" since in a higher concentration it will be irritating. One or two drops of peppermint added to a bath is wonderfully cooling; however more than that is too cold.

Peppermint may be either cooling or warming depending on the dilution used. In low dilutions (less than 2%), it is very cooling. In high dilutions, greater then 5%, it will be warming (a rubifactant) and serve as a counter-irritant in pain relief blends. Applied topically in low dilution, it is an excellent headache remedy.

Blends with: black pepper, fennel, ginger, lemon, lemongrass, and rosemary

WARNING: Peppermint cools by constricting the capillaries and needs to be used in extremely low dilutions. It is also an irritant. One or two drops in a bath is sufficient, use a 1% dilution for massage or other skin applications. Also, recent research indicates that the use of peppermint essential oil may aggravate GERD (gastroesophageal reflux disease-type of heart burn). It is contraindicated in cases of gallbladder inflammation.

PINE, Scotch *Pinus sylvestris*

Parts used: Needles—steam distilled

True Scotch pine is a delightful essential oil. Many commercial distillers (and vendors), however, are apt to label any combination of any pine species *Pinus sylvestris*. Perhaps that explains why so many "pine" samples smell like bathroom cleaners. In truth, pure Scotch pine is a rare oil, not to be limited to cleaning bathrooms.

Physically, all pine oils are antiseptic, antifungal, and detoxifying. For detoxifying, use it in a sauna. It enters the body through inhalation and expels toxins through perspiration. A few drops of pine and either lemon or lemon eucalyptus in a scrub bucket will cleanse all surfaces, aiding in the elimination of unwanted bacteria and fungi on floors, in the tub, etc. It's a good addition to any cleaning mix. For coughs, colds, and congestion, add pine, eucalyptus, and lavender to the diffuser. Pine is an excellent expectorant, helping release mucous and ease breathing. It can help clear congestion in the sinuses, lungs, and bronchial passages. (For this purpose, I'd think about a steam inhalation, rather than a diffuser, the moisture of the steam will compliment the effects of the pine.)

Blends with: eucalyptus, ginger, spike lavender, lemon, lemongrass, and rosemary

WARNING: Pine oil can be irritating to the skin; I prefer to use it in an airborne blend, rather than in the bath or on the skin. It should be avoided by those with allergies.

ROSE OTTO *Rosa damascena*

Parts used: Petals—hydro distilled

Rose otto (rose essential oil) is produced in many countries. The only ones worth investing in are produced in Bulgaria or Turkey. Those produced in other countries simply are not of the same quality, and, although less expensive, will not give you the value of true rose otto. The ultimate woman's oil, rose is calming and supportive. Rose oil is believed by many to help balance female hormones, regulate the menstrual cycle, and ease the discomforts of PMS and menopause. Rose oil is helpful to all skin types, but excels in blends for mature skin. Rose has no parallel in treating grief, hysteria, or depression.

Mix with frankincense to ease heartache. A touch of rose is a must in any aphrodisiac blend. I find that sandalwood and rose can make a wonderful romantic blend for both men and women. For the man, use mostly sandalwood oil with just a touch of rose otto; for the woman, use mostly rose with just a touch of sandalwood.

If you are wanting the rose oil strictly for scent, please try rose absolute; it does smell more like a fresh cut rose, however the presence of the solvents used to produce it make the absolute less appropriate for healing. Undiluted rose otto can become solid at a cool room temperature. If this happens to yours, you can roll the bottle around in your hand for a few minutes, or put it in some warm water, and it will liquefy. Rose will tend to overwhelm any other oil used in blends. Start with perhaps one drop of rose oil to perhaps 10 drops of the oils you want to blend it with. The rose will still be noticeable even at a very low percentage.

Blends with: frankincense, jasmine, lemongrass, mandarin, patchouli, sandalwood, and vetiver

ROSE ABSOLUTE (Rose Maroc)
Rosa damascena or Rosa centifolia

Parts used: Flowers—solvent extracted

The use of solvents yields a deeper, richer rose aroma, making the absolute far better for perfumery, and perhaps for emotional uses. However, for skin care, for internal uses, and for physical effects, the pure steam distilled rose otto is the wiser choice. Both are well worth experiencing. One luxury-loving client recommends blending the two for the ultimate sensory experience. The absolute is a deep orange in color, and needs diluting to be truly appreciated. Because solvent extraction produces more absolute than the hydro distillation used to produce true rose otto, the absolute should be less costly.

Blends with: frankincense, jasmine, lemongrass, mandarin, patchouli, sandalwood, and vetiver

ROSEMARY OILS *Rosemary officinalis*

Parts used: Flowering tops—steam distilled

The culinary herb rosemary has three different chemotypes that yield very different essential oils, with different uses. I'd not use any rosemary in the evening; it is far too stimulating and ruins my sleep. Also, avoid using if you are pregnant, have high blood pressure, or if you have a diagnosed seizure disorder.

Blends with: All three rosemary oils blend well with basil, bergamot, black pepper, cedarwood, citronella, cypress, eucalyptus, ginger, juniper, hyssop, lavender, lavandin, lemon, marjoram, mints, origanum, pine needle, olibanum, petitgrain, sage, tea tree, and vetiver.

ROSEMARY Camphor (Spanish Rosemary) *Rosemarinus officinalis var Camphor*

Parts used: Leaves and flowering tops—steam distilled

If you are looking for the old fashioned traditional high-in-camphor rosemary oil to use in decongestive or pain relief blends, this should be your choice. It is strongly camphorous in aroma, but for some uses, is the best choice. For example, rosemary camphor has been proven to be a strong antispasmodic, so would be useful in easing muscle cramps, rheumatism, poor circulation, and perhaps intestinal cramping.

ROSEMARY Cineole
Rosemarinus officinalis var Cineole

Parts used: Flowers and leaves—steamed distilled

Wonderfully fresh and stimulating, rosemary cineole is known for its ability to wake up the body and spirit. In a massage oil, it can stimulate circulation, and it is often used in blends for cellulite and edema. In cosmetics and soaps, it is believed to combat acne, dandruff, and excessively oily skin. A drop added to shampoo makes dark hair glow, and may stimulate hair growth. Rosemary cineole is said to be useful in treating respiratory conditions, especially those stemming from nervous or emotional causes, such as many forms of asthma.

ROSEMARY Verbenon
Rosemarinus officianalis var Verbenon

Parts used: Flowering tops—steam distilled

Gentler and less stimulating than our more traditional cineole rich rosemary, this chemotype is most frequently recommended for skin care. Rosemary verbenon is recommended by many authorities for its cellular regenerative powers. I have frequently seen rosemary verbenon recommended for the treatment of oily skin and scalp and dandruff. In my experience, this lovely chemotype lacks the stimulating effects of most rosemary oils, which makes it much more appropriate for adding to an evening shower or shampoo. I find it relaxing, rather than stimulating. Put on a CD of ocean sounds, add one drop of seaweed essential oil and five or six drops of this lovely rosemary, and perhaps a touch of fennel to a bath, lean back, relax, and experience the ocean. Verbenon is a ketone which could be toxic in high doses. For this reason, avoid in pregnancy, with babies, or children.

SANDALWOOD *Santalum album India*

Parts used: Wood—steam distilled

While there are other varieties of sandalwood, grown in other geographic areas, none of them have the aromatic splendor of true Indian sandalwood. Indian sandalwood is an endangered species. The oil is very rare and export is often banned by the Indian government. For this reason, many refuse to use it. This rich and sweet scented oil is known as an aid to meditation and as an aphrodisiac. Sandalwood essential oil acts as a tonic to the immune system, and is often used in treating urinary tract problems. It balances both dry and oily skin, is useful in treating acne, and is helpful in soothing barber's rash. Emotionally, it relaxes stress, soothes irritation, and lifts depression. Keep in mind that sandalwood is somewhat thick and may have a hard time coming out of the orifice reducer. It may be necessary to pipette the oil out. Sandalwood oil, properly stored, will only improve with age. Buy what you need for today, but invest in enough to last you over the coming decades. Sandalwood is known as the universal blender, since very few aromatics do not blend well with its smooth softness.

Blends with: 'Atlas' cedarwood, benzoin, neroli, orange and all the sweeter citrus oils, patchouli, vanilla, and rose

SPRUCE, Black *Picea mariana*

Parts used: Wild needles—steam distilled

Emotionally, I find black spruce freeing, uplifting, and mentally stimulating. My resources recommend it for mental and physical exhaustion as well as for relief of both stress and anxiety. I have seen it recommended for muscle aches and pains, aching joints, poor circulation, and muscle spasms.

It also could be helpful for bronchitis or asthma. I've found that a blend of black spruce, clary and a touch of Bulgarian lavender is just wonderful in an end of the day bath blend—the cares and tensions of the day disappear.

TEA TREE *Melaleuca alternifolia*

Parts used: Leaves—steam distilled

Tea tree has won a reputation as a cure-all because of its powerful antifungal, antiviral, and antibacterial properties. It is the first suggestion for athlete's foot, nail viruses, and other fungal infections. Often used in anti-acne remedies, as well as in a diffuser to combat the flu and other viral infections. It is often recommended as the remedy for a vaginal candida infection.

Blends with: 'Atlas' cedarwood, bergamot, black pepper, ginger, and lavender

TEA TREE, Lemon *Leptospermon petersonii*

Parts used: Leaves—steam distilled

This relatively unknown Australian essential oil has two valuable attributes. First, when blended with the "traditional" tea tree (*Melaleuca alternifolia*, above) it has been shown to heighten the antibacterial effects. Together, they form a more powerful antibacterial synergy than either oil used alone. Lemon tea tree is also known as a powerful natural repellant for mosquitoes and other insect repellants.

VETIVER *Vetivera zizanoides*

Parts used: Roots—hydro distilled

Honey textured and colored, this thickest of essential oils is the perfect base oil to anchor a blend. I use it to smooth and sweeten some of my blends, since vetiver is less apt to "take over" a blend than some of the other base notes. Emotionally, vetiver is very grounding and balancing. Vetiver is a key ingredient in anti-anxiety blends. I use it daily blended with neroli, petitgrain, and a touch of citrus. It balances sebum production, so is useful in treating both oily and dry skin. Vetiver is far too thick to come out of the largest orifice reducers. When you receive a bottle of it, you will need to remove the reducer and pipette, or pour the oil out. Be sure to replace the reducer when you're done as it creates a seal between the bottle and cap. Vetiver is perfect in any blend that needs a sweet base note to anchor it.

Blends with: jasmine, neroli, orange, patchouli, petitgrain, and rose

YLANG-YLANG *Cananga odorafa*

fractionally distilled

Ylang-ylang is the one essential oil that is always distilled in "fractions." This means that the distillation is stopped at various stages, with the essential oil taken off at each stage. Various "grades" of ylang-ylang are thus produced. Each distiller makes his own determination of where the "dividing line" should be, so there is a wide range of quality from one distiller to another. The normal production will include ylang-ylang extra, and ylang-ylang 1, 2, and 3.

Ylang-ylang is known in Asia as an antidepressant, relaxing to body, mind, and spirit. It is said to calm anger, release tension, lift depression and generally stabilize mood swings. It is also used as an aphrodisiac. Physically, it has been used to lower blood pressure, ease muscle spasms and muscles tension, and treat PMS and menopausal symptoms. In a facial oil or cream, it can help balance sebum production and is most helpful to oily skin. It also can fight the bacteria that often contribute to acne. Ylang-ylang is said to stimulate hair growth and might be a useful addition to a shampoo or conditioner.

Blends with: bergamot, lavender, lemon, narcissus, neroli, palma rosa, sandalwood, and vetiver